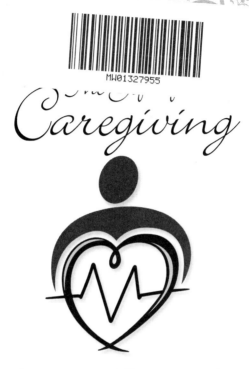

Caregiving

Daily Inspirations, Affirmations and Tips

Rebecca Sharp Colmer
EKLEKTIKA Press, Inc.
Chelsea, MI

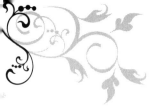

©2011 Rebecca Sharp Colmer
EKLEKTIKA Press, Inc.
PO Box 157
Chelsea, MI 48118

All rights reserved. No part of this book may reproduced or transmitted in any form by any means, electronic or mechanical, including photocopying, recording, or by any information storage or retrieval system, without written permission from the author.

Copyright 2011 by Rebecca Sharp Colmer

Library of Congress Card No. 2011923685

ISBN: 978-0-9823250-2-5

Printed in the United States of America

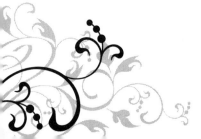

With Gratitude

Dear _____ ,
(caregiver's name)

This book is dedicated to you. You have an important and challenging job.
Thank you for helping to take care of

_____ .
(care-receiver's name)

Your time, caring and generosity is greatly appreciated.

Sincerely,

_____

Introduction

The caregiver role is complex and differs for everyone depending on the needs of the care-receiver. I have found that words can inspire, motivate, and even change us if we let them.

May this book be an inspiration for you when and as you need it, no matter where you are in the process of caregiving. Repeat the daily affirmations aloud. May you know peace, kindness, and love.

Best wishes, RSC

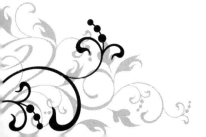

January 1 - Possibilities

Today, anything is possible. We accept the conditions presently in our lives. On this first day of the year we believe we will be happy, healthy, strong, and compassionate as the days and weeks unfold.

Each day is a new beginning. We will set realistic goals and work hard as we resolve to maintain good care practices in the coming months.

Today is full of possibilities. Today I believe in myself.

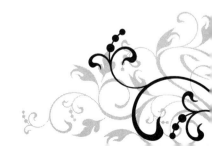

January 2 - Positive Affirmations

Just as other people's words affect us, the words we say to ourselves also affect our attitude. Whether we feel negative or positive depends on the input we get, including the input we get from ourselves.

Using positive affirmations is a proven technique that works miracles in many lives.

Don't be shy. Repeat the affirmation, out loud, at the bottom of each page.

I discipline myself to do the things I need to do.

January 3 - Health

A good dose of fresh air helps to promote motivation and perseverance. However, in the winter months it is often too cold and during the summer months it's often too hot or humid for us to want to be outside. We end up with a lack of fresh oxygen!

It's our responsibility to find a way to get better quality air — the kind that encourages cheerfulness and motivation.

I choose to be healthy and free. I will go outside every day of the year.

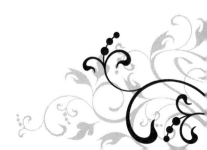

January 4 - Laughter

Laughter reduces our stress levels. Laughter provides a physical and emotional release. Laughter takes the focus away from anger, guilt, stress and negative emotions in a more complete way than mere distractions.

Practice smiling and laughing. You may be surprised that real smiles, genuine laughter and merriment may follow.

Today, I will not take myself too seriously. I will smile every day.

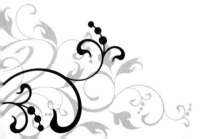

January 5 - Self Control

We only have control over three things in life. They are:
- Our thoughts.
- The images we visualize.
- Our behavior (the actions we take).

Most of us are stuck in our conditioned responses and end up being run by our habits so that we never change our behavior.

If we don't like what we are producing and experiencing, we have to change our responses and habits.

I will give up blaming and complaining.

January 6 - Breathing

When we are facing a stressful situation, we can reduce stress by deep breathing. Try this: sit comfortably with your back straight. Put one hand on your chest and the other on your stomach. Inhale through your nose and the hand on your stomach should begin to rise. Your other hand shouldn't move very much. Exhale as much air as you can by contracting your stomach muscles.

I will practice deep breathing several times every day.

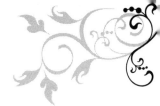

January 7 - Fear

Many caregivers are fearful of how others will judge them. We all have periods of self-doubt and discouragement about ourselves, ranging from lack of confidence in our skills to discomfort with our impatience and attitude.

Only by recognizing and understanding these fears can we overcome their negative effects on our performance. We need to think about how they originate and how realistic they are. Most of the time, we are our own toughest critic.

Today I will acknowledge my fears and confront them.

January 8 - Attitude

"Fake it till you make it. Act as if." It is important to behave the way we want to be, even though we don't really feel it yet. In time, we will feel the magic. Our good attitude will be rewarded with a positive mental state.

The attitude we cultivate (whether good or bad) will determine how the daily events in our lives affect us.

My good attitude will make this a great day.

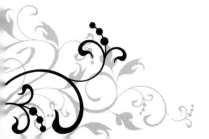

January 9 - Reactions

Mastering our reactions is a good stress management technique for our loved-one or patient; and it leaves us feeling calm and in control.

Slow, deep breathing is important when people are feeling anxious. When we are stressed, breathing often becomes rapid and shallow, resulting in an increased heart rate that the brain might interpret as a further increase in anxiety.

Before reacting today I will pause and make a thoughtful and responsible choice.

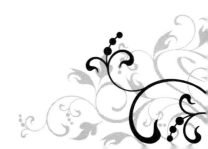

January 10 - Happiness

Happiness is within our power. It lives within all of us even though sometimes we can't seem to find it.

We must practice tapping into this source within us, regardless of our circumstances. Too often we look outside ourselves for the key to happiness. We look in all the wrong places — food, alcohol, drugs.

Take a moment to smile and be happy.

Happiness is my birthright. I will share a smile with everyone I meet today.

January 11 - Creativity

We may think that being a caregiver day in and day out leaves little room for being creative. In fact, to be powerful in life, we have to take the position that we create, or allow, everything that happens to us.

Successful caregivers face facts squarely. We do the uncomfortable and take steps to create our desired outcomes. We make things happen.

I feel great. I am in control. I will make things happen.

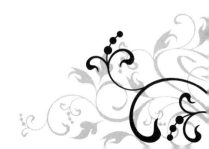

January 12 - Feedback

Once we begin to take action, we start getting feedback about whether we are doing the right thing. Once we receive feedback we have to be willing to adjust our actions if necessary.

As caregivers we shouldn't be afraid to ask for corrective feedback from our care-receiver.

Next, we have to listen to the feedback and determine if it is accurate. Is there a pattern? Do we need to make a course correction?

I will receive and respond to feedback.

January 13 - Communication

Gaining the cooperation and help of family members can make our caregiving job easier. Being able to articulate our feelings and needs will help our family members help us.

Communication within families is special and unique. Good communication requires both good speaking and good listening skills.

We can improve our chances of being heard if we use "*I*" statements rather than "*you*" statements which may be interpreted as blaming statements.

I will listen attentively. I will listen respectfully.

January 14 - Stress

Caregivers are often surprised at some of the negative feelings we have. If any of these feelings are judged as unacceptable, there may be an unconscious tendency to try and hide them. If they are masked or hidden they become major contributors to stress.

By changing our thoughts we can change the way we feel and respond to any situation. We can learn to modify our feelings since they are a by-product of thoughts and messages we send to ourselves.

I will explore my feelings and defenses. I will share my feelings with someone I trust.

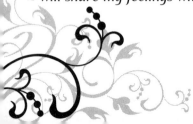

January 15 - Gratitude

When we feel drained or depleted from caregiving we can quickly change our energy level by looking at the good things we have and saying thanks — thank you self, thank you God.

Whatever we appreciate and give thanks for will actually increase in our life. Gratitude and thanks are a path straight to the heart, to our essence and soul.

Gratitude is healing to our emotions.

I will express my appreciation of my loved-one/patient, to him or her.

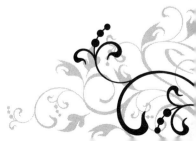

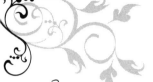

January 16 - Action

One of the most difficult aspects of the caregiver role is that the job continues seven days a week, 24 hours a day. Many times every day we are called upon to take action.

Our actions reveal who we are, to ourselves and others. Giving it our best shot is what counts. If we can honestly say that we have made a 100 percent effort, then no matter what the outcome, we can be proud of ourselves.

If I don't give up or give in, I'll have no regrets because I will have given my all.

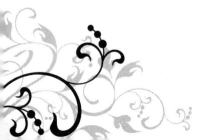

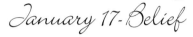

January 17 - Belief

Today, anything is possible. We have to believe that we are great caregivers.

It feels good to have self-confidence and the desire to enhance our caregiving skills, strength and stamina.

We have to believe that we can we handle any situation that comes up.

I love who I am and all that I do. I believe I am guided to be a success.

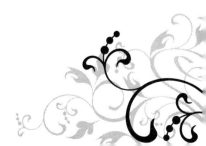

January 18 - Teamwork

We can't do our caregiving job without the help of others. The way the team works as a whole determines its success. We must be careful not to become too wrapped up in our own performance at the expense of the care-receiver and the rest of the team.

As members of the care team, we must learn to share the work, the glory, and the disappointments. We can't do it alone.

I will share the care. I will encourage others to be a part of our team.

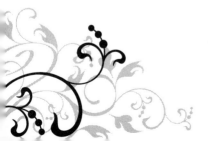

January 19 - Preparation

When we are prepared, we are more confident and comfortable. In addition to having a care plan for our loved-one/patient, we need a strategic plan for ourselves.

We need to set up our plan to include personal goals, targets, and rewards. Preparation is the key to enjoying ourselves and reducing stress. Preparation is also vital to success in our endeavors.

We shouldn't mindlessly perform our job without a plan.

I will review my plan and improve my strategy today.

January 20 - Respite

If we begin to feel overworked or over-obligated it may be time to take a break or vary our routine.

Respite care is important because it reduces the incidence of caregiver burnout. Respite care is temporary care given by another in place of the primary caregiver so the primary caregiver can take a break. When we rest for a few minutes, a few hours, or a few days, when we begin again, we can start fresh and be reminded of the joy in our job.

I will take a break. I will be driven by compassion and not obligation.

January 21 - Confidence

We can keep our confidence healthy by taking a close look at our caregiving abilities. We need to step back and assess where we are and where we have been. A check of our past accomplishments can do wonders when we are feeling insecure. We know that we can achieve what we set our hearts on.

We have a right to be confident. We work hard and strive to meet our goals and make progress every day.

I am confident in my abilities and in myself. I've earned my rewards.

January 22 - Visualization

If we don't have a caregiving plan, we put our patient/care-receiver at risk. Part of the planning process involves actually picturing what we are going to do.

Visualization is a dress rehearsal so that we can work out any kinks before we actually run into them.

When we are visualizing, we have the advantage because we can always imagine being successful.

I will rehearse in my mind before I go to work today.

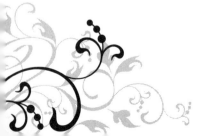

January 23 - Pressure

Pressure (or stress) can crush us or it can lift us up and inspire us. Pressure can come from the outside—our loved-one/patient, the doctors, or family members. Pressure can also come from within.

Pressure can also help us to rise to the occasion and work harder than we ever thought possible. Sometimes positive stress can contribute to a better focus. When handled appropriately, pressure can get us on track as nothing else can.

I will make the pressure work for me today.

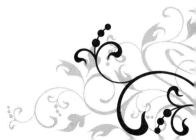

January 24 - Positive Attitude

Staying up when we are feeling low, or looking forward to another caregiving day with enthusiasm — instead of doom and gloom — may not be easy — but it will be worth it in the long run.

The energy spent on anger, frustration, or insecurity is better spent on concentration, perseverance, and affirmation.

An upbeat attitude can take us a long way.

I will keep a positive attitude today.

January 25 - Moderation

We all overdo from time to time. We go out and push ourselves to the limit. Overdoing it can lead to sickness, disappointment, and even burnout.

Moderation is the best approach. It's much more important to keep working steadily, than to make what may seem like great strides all at once.

One of the easiest ways to practice moderation is to share the care and ask for help.

I will not overdo. I will ask for help.

January 26 - Flexibility

Super-rigid caregiving plans are very susceptible to falling apart. The more inflexible we are, the more likely we are to run into disappointment. Adapting to the situation at hand can mean the difference between a good day and a bad day.

Flexibility can also help us to become more rounded. We'll find that if we are willing to adapt our daily tasks we will be more successful.

Today I will be less rigid.

January 27 - Patience

Patience is a virtue. Patience. Patience. Patience.

Not being patient will eventually lead to frustration. If we cut ourselves some slack we will feel the benefits both mentally and emotionally.

We have to believe that we can take care of our loved-one/patient, no matter the situation. If we approach our loved-one with patience, we will find out that we'll enjoy them a lot more.

Every situation is an opportunity for me to practice patience.

January 28 - Exercise

No matter how spun up we may be, no matter how stressful some relationships may be, we can always benefit from some exercise. Without fail, a brief walk can do us a world of good.

More than a drink or a smoke, exercise is the most consistent way to soothe the mind and body.

When we are under pressure, our shoulders are tense, our brains are clogged, it is now time to blow it out with a brisk walk.

I will take a walk today.

January 29 - Forgiveness

In order to move on we have to let go. In the world of family caregiving we need to come from a place of love and forgiveness. Hanging on to past hurts is incompatible with caregiving.

When we forgive it puts us back in the present. When we learn whatever lesson is presented and move on we are no longer wasting valuable energy.

I release myself from all the hurt that has kept me limited.

January 30 - Grief

The collective weight of losses that accumulate over a lifetime can burden us in powerful and painful ways.

It is important to realize the grieving process is something that both the care-receiver and caregiver will experience.

We grieve spouses, parents, siblings, and friends. We grieve lost opportunities. We grieve lost hope for the future.

I will reminisce about good times.

January 31 - Time Management

In order to be a successful caregiver in achieving our goals and creating our desired atmosphere, we have to get good at saying no to the people and distractions that can derail us.

Successful caregivers know how to say no without feeling guilty. We have to eliminate tasks, requests, and other time-stealers that don't have a high payoff for our loved-one/patient.

Today I will only answer emails that are truly important.

February 1 - Laughter

Laughter is not only fun and contagious, but may be one of the healthiest things we can do. Laughter is a form of catharsis that provides an outlet for feelings of stress and anxiety.

Laughter helps relax tense muscles. Laughter helps the body produce new immune cells faster. Laughter helps our brain to release endorphins.

I will find five things to laugh at today.

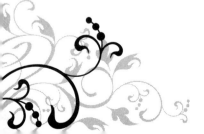

February 2 - Feelings

In the busy-ness of our everyday life, we may not set aside the time to ponder our deeper feelings about the person for whom we are providing care.

Try keeping a journal or diary. Even just writing down our feelings on a sheet of paper can be very healing because it allows us to express what is really inside of us.

My work is a joy and a pleasure. I will explore my feelings daily.

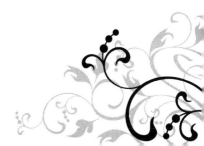

February 3 - Friendships

Maintaining the close relationships we have formed in our lives gives us a sense of well-being and support. Our true friends accept us, warts and all.

It is important for our well-being to continue our friendships rather than let them go because of the demands of caregiving.

Caregivers who give up close relationships that are meaningful to them are at a greater risk for depression, isolation, and health problems.

I will call my best friend today and schedule a time to get together.

February 4 - Imperfection

Many caregivers think they must do everything perfectly. No one does everything perfectly. Caregiving is a learning process that changes from day to day. We need to give ourselves permission to learn as we go, and even make mistakes along the way.

If we have put forth our best effort, we should be proud of our achievements, even though the road may not always be smooth.

I am proud each and every time I give my best effort.

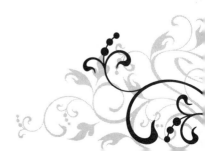

February 5 - Perspective

Daily caregiving can cause us to overreact, blow things out of proportion, and even hold on too tightly. If we get paralyzed by little things when we are irritated or annoyed, our reactions can actually get in the way of delivering good care.

If we lose sight of the bigger picture and focus on the negative, we may end up annoying and alienating other people who might otherwise help us.

I will replace old habits of reaction with new habits of perspective.

February 6 - Serenity

The serenity prayer suggests, *"Change the things that can be changed, accept those that cannot, and have the wisdom to know the difference."* When we learn to *"let go"* of problems instead of resisting with all our might, life will get easier.

Learning to respond to life gracefully helps us to create a more peaceful and loving caregiving situation.

I will let go of the "small stuff" today.

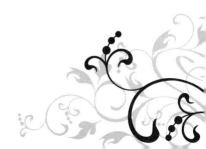

February 7 - Inner Peace

When we have inner peace, we are less distracted by our wants, desires, and concerns. It is much easier to concentrate and focus on taking care of our loved-one or patient.

When we are fearful or wound up we are prevented from attaining our greatest potential. We can accomplish just as much while being relaxed, peaceful and loving.

I will slow down today. I will relax, knowing that I will still do a great job.

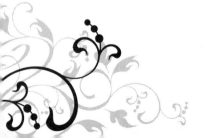

February 8 - Self-care

In the business world there is an old adage that you must pay yourself first. The same principle needs to be implemented into our caregiving practice.

We should schedule a little time each day for ourselves, as if it were an actual appointment. In the long run we will be happier, healthier and better caregivers.

We can find the time we need for ourselves.

Today I will take some time to read and reflect on myself.

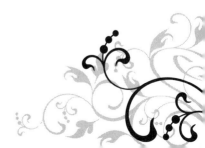

February 9 - Power

Our thoughts are very powerful. In order to experience a feeling we must first have a thought that produces that feeling.

The next time we are upset we need to remind ourselves that it is our thinking that is negative and not our life. This simple exercise will be the first step in putting us back on the path to happiness.

Practice thinking of negative thoughts in the same way you would treat flies at a picnic. You shoo them away and get on with your enjoyment.

My thoughts are powerful. I will capitalize on positive thoughts.

February 10 - Reflection

Keep a journal. Personal reflection of our caregiving experiences, along with self-initiated feedback can boost motivation. We should write down our feelings, concerns, dreams, progress, and private thoughts.

If we review our journal often, we will gain an appreciation for our progress. Being totally honest about our feelings will help us to focus our efforts while reminding us we may need to tend to our stress.

The more I understand, the more my world expands.

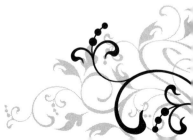

February 11 - Positive Friendships

Good stress can help compel us to action while bad stress can result in feelings of anger, rejection, distrust, and depression.

We should surround ourselves with friends who *"think positive."* We are all susceptible to the beliefs, values, and attitudes of our peers.

It is important that we spend more time with those who are optimistic and motivated, especially if our loved-one/patient has a negative attitude.

I am supported by good friends. I will share my joy.

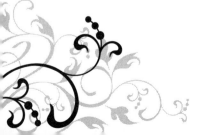

February 12 - Obstacles

When starting the day, we should troubleshoot our tasks and analyze up front any potential roadblocks, hazards, or uncertainties. What possible negative factors will arise?

Lack of support, knowledge, time, physical space, energy, money, or experience can make the task seem daunting.

Handle as many of these obstacles as early as possible. Then we will feel more positive about our chances of success.

I will go over, around or through any obstacle I encounter.

February 13 - Planning

Always create a *"Plan B"*. Even if we totally expect to succeed, we need a back-up plan. What will we do if things don't fall into place? If others don't come through? If we get sick? If the weather becomes horrible?

With an alternate plan we can relax in the knowledge that even in the worst case scenario, we will be all right.

I make back up plans that are beneficial to me and my care-receiver/patient.

February 14 - Positive Attitude

We should attach positive values to each of our caregiving tasks. If we have to clean up the living room, realize that the accomplishment of the project will make us feel good about our living area. If we have to update personal health records, associate it with saving money while improving health.

If we have to call a friend to discuss an uncomfortable situation, think of it as a means of gaining courage, reducing stress, and building a greater trust.

Every task I do has a positive outcome.

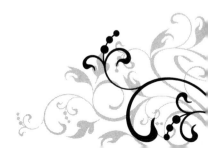

February 15 - Love

We are here to love and be loved, both caregivers and care-receivers. Love rewards us by bringing meaning to our lives.

The greatest truth is love. Love will guide us to the solution for every problem we encounter. Look for the love in every situation.

Whatever my problem is today, the solution is love.

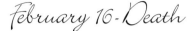

February 16 - Death

At some point it becomes clear that our loved-one/patient is not immortal despite the best efforts of the care team.

We are all going to die. It is a normal and natural process. Death is not a failure. It is a process, the final stage of living. It demands both practical and emotional involvement.

Acknowledge the process and celebrate life.

The love we share greets us in our next experience.

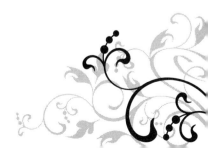

February 17 - Challenges

Becoming a caregiver is a big undertaking and it doesn't come with a specific job description.

Often the role of caregiving is unexpected and comes at a time when we are unprepared. Keep in mind that even the most prepared caregivers face new challenges every day.

All my experiences are part of the richness and fullness of my life.

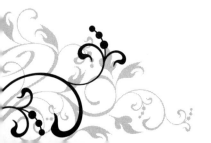

February 18 – Kindness

When we are kind to others, we become kinder. It doesn't take much to be nice, flash a smile, give a pat on the shoulder. When we commit these simple acts of kindness we set in motion a positive domino effect.

When we improve another's life in a small but not insignificant way, that person is more likely to reach out and do the same.

I will practice random acts of kindness today.

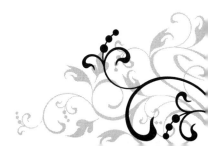

February 19 - Overcoming

Pressure is often a true test of our commitment and motivation. Caregivers who throw in the towel at the first sign of a little opposition or difficulty won't get very far.

A little bit of pressure can help to bring out the best in us. Heart is the ability to rise to any occasion, no matter what the circumstances, day in and day out.

Resist giving in, keep on fighting.

Pressure will enhance my job, not hurt it.

February 20 - Tenacity

Tenacity backed with faith in ourselves is an almost unbeatable combination and is the ideal ingredient in the formula for successful caregiving.

Our belief in what we can accomplish will take us to a certain level of care, and it will help us to continue to improve and grow. Add in a "never say quit" attitude and we will consistently be armed for success.

I am confident. I never give up.

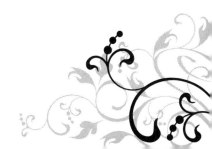

February 21 - Experience

There is no such thing as an overnight expert. At first we will spend time working on the basics. No matter how tedious it feels, it is time well spent. Eventually we will be able to grow beyond the basics.

We become better caregivers every day as we face new experiences and challenges. One day, we will know we are an experienced caregiver and know we can handle any situation that arises.

I will put in the time and reap the rewards of experience.

February 22 - Relieving Stress

To be our best, we need to release tension and keep ourselves as flexible as possible — both physically and mentally. If we are all wound up, we will not be able to perform our caregiving duties well and we will make mistakes.

It is important to keep our nerves under control. If we let them take over then our anxiety is dictating how we will perform.

Jumping up and down or doing some quick exercises will help burn off nervous energy. Breathing deeply can also be helpful.

I'll relax before my nerves threaten to take over.

February 23 - Anxiety

No matter who we are or how much experience we have, chances are there will be times when we will be nervous about our job. The key is to not let this feeling distract us but to recognize it, accept it, and try to use it to our advantage.

While it can be hard to ward off nervousness once it hits, by acknowledging it and trying to channel this extra energy into our efforts we can often make use of this potentially debilitating feeling.

When I feel anxious, I will recognize the feeling and channel it positively.

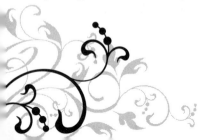

February 24 - Expectations

Expectations, like goals are important in caregiving. They give us something to strive for, something to push toward. By expecting something of ourselves, we are setting a minimum at which we believe we can perform.

While it is important to keep expectations in check—not too high and therefore reachable—it is helpful to keep adjusting them upward to encourage improvement.

I will adjust my expectations as my experience grows.

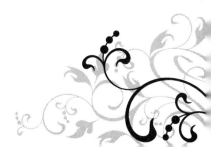

February 25 - Support

Caregiver support helps us to see that our situation is not unique, that others face many of the same difficult issues and feelings. This in itself can be a big relief.

Call someone that you haven't spoken to in a while. Tell them about your caregiving experiences. Ask them to do you a favor. Ask them to check in on you.

This kind of peer support can do wonders.

I will reach out to an old friend.

February 26 - Praise

Just as you praise children for developing new skills, praise your loved-one/patient when he or she tries a new task or makes steps to be independent.

Being a good cheerleader will help both the care-receiver and the caregiver. It is important to help our patient/care-receiver when they absolutely need it. But it is also important to let them care for themselves, others and the world around them.

Today I will not do "too much" for my loved-one.

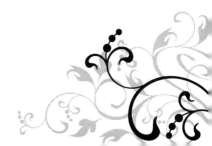

February 27 - Blessings

Regardless of how many things go wrong or how hard we must struggle for small successes, most of us are blessed.

If we make a list (written or mental) of all the things we have to be grateful for, this may be all it takes to put things in the proper perspective.

I am blessed to be hardworking and honest. I am blessed to be able to take care of my loved-one.

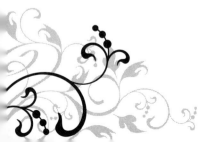

February 28 - Strengths

Each caregiver and family must understand their own strengths and their unique set of problems. If our health and well-being is threatened, our loved-ones are in jeopardy. As caregivers we must see ourselves as valuable, important, and worthy of the time necessary to meet our own needs, or those whom we care for will suffer.

A higher strength empowers me to move ahead with courage and determination.

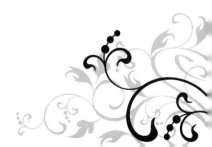

February 29 - Guilt

Many caregivers have strong guilt feelings because they are unable to help their loved-one get well. One of the most important things we can do is to recognize that our health and worth must be as highly valued as the health and worth of our loved-one.

We must give ourselves credit for our accomplishments and judge ourselves, *"Not Guilty"*, and accept the very best that life can provide for us.

I will live in the present and enjoy the moment.

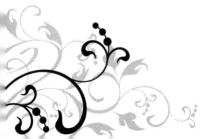

March 1 - Compliments

We can spark our creative caregiving energy by positive self-talk. Each us can be our own one-person cheerleading squad.

To get started, stand in front of the mirror and repeat the following:

Outstanding. Excellent. Fantastic. Exceptional. Unrivaled. Incredible. Nurturing. Notable. Amazing. Fabulous. Impressive. Grand. Beautiful. Loving. Spectacular. Remarkable. Wonderful. Kind. Extraordinary. Splendid. Impressive.

Today I will find the words to compliment myself.

March 2 - Friendship

By fostering a friendship approach to giving care, we encourage reciprocal and empowering interactions with our care-receivers. Friendship requires getting to know a person well, desiring what is best for the other, feeling sympathy and empathy, being honest and trustworthy.

We should treat the people in our care as a friend and in the same way we would like to be treated.

Today I will offer my care-receiver true friendship.

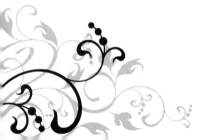

March 3 - Imagination

Imagination not only helps to increase our happiness, it also helps us to achieve what we want out of life. Reactivate those childlike centers in our minds.

Harnessing our imagination and our skills of observation can help us to reclaim this lost way of seeing.

We should allow ourselves a little time to daydream and wander.

I am happy because I imagine it so.

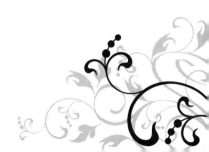

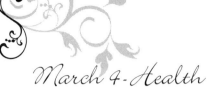

March 4 - Health

Aerobic exercise is one of the best ways to stay healthy. Aim for at least 20 minutes a day.

Aerobic exercise reduces muscle tension and the amount of stress hormones in the body. It also boosts endorphins and releases additional serotonin in the brain, which helps to balance our mood and relieve depression.

A brisk walk or a short bicycle ride is all it takes!

Today I will increase my heart rate through moderate exercise.

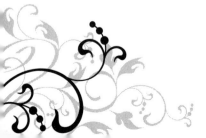

March 5 - Breathing

The way we breathe affects our mental state. When we hyperventilate — breathing rapidly in reaction to a stressful situation or frightening moment — we put ourselves into a hard-to-break cycle, because the quick breathing doesn't allow enough oxygen to reach our brain. That, in turn, can make us feel even more anxious.

When we concentrate on our breathing, we are better able to remain present in the moment instead of thinking anxiously about what is coming next.

I will practice slow, deep breathing, five times today.

March 6 - Information

Caregivers need complete information about their loved-one/patient's diagnosis or disease — in layman's terms. We need answers to questions and an opportunity to learn what to expect as the condition progresses.

We should not hesitate to ask that issues be restated or clarified when necessary.

I will write down my questions and concerns so I can get answers.

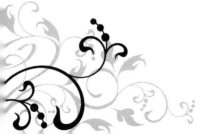

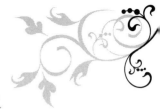

March 7 - Grief

Family members need time to grieve with the one who is ill. With progressive dementia, this is only possible in the early stages. During this time, family members may want to mend fences, do things that have been put off *"until a more convenient time"* and say the loving things that are often postponed until too late.

Today I will say "I love you."

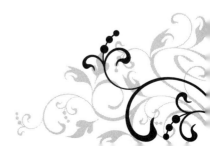

March 8 - Counseling

Caregivers often benefit from individual and small group counseling services which concentrate on feelings, identification, stress management techniques, and strengthening the family.

Professional help at various levels of disease progression may benefit both the care-receiver and the caregiver.

I will ask for help today. I will share my feelings.

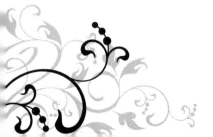

March 9 - End-of-Life Issues

Most families want to consider independent living for their loved-one for as long as possible. However, it is important to develop resources for intermediate assistance, complete nursing care, and preparation for death. Decisions regarding living wills, regular wills, and funeral preferences will need to be made.

I am prepared. I will review our options.

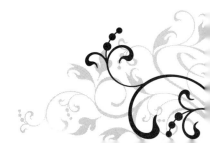

March 10 - Consequences of Stress

It is very important that we take care of ourselves as we care for our loved-one, watching for any signals of stress that our bodies may be sending. If we become ill, who will care for us?

Our loved-one's demands on our time, our combined feelings of grief, anger, love, and frustration, and all our other unrelated responsibilities far exceed healthy boundaries. Caregivers often feel powerless over this situation, which can lead to more stress.

I change my life when I reduce my stress.

March 11 - Work Load

Caregivers should never attempt to *"go it alone."* We will eventually break, and the burden will become infinitely greater for everyone involved.

It is necessary to build a network of substitute caregivers who will assist with miscellaneous tasks on a regular basis. This may be possible through a combination of family members, friends, church or social groups, or public agencies that provide respite care.

I will share the care today.

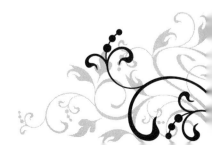

March 12 - Change

Dementia caregivers must realize that as our loved-one's brain deteriorates, even the most basic skills will be lost.

One day our patient will function fairly well, and on the next a simple task becomes impossible. Insisting that he or she do certain tasks will frustrate him/her and make the symptoms worse.

I am gentle and patient.

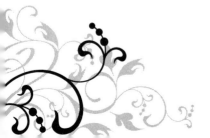

March 13 - Affection

As caregivers, we can enhance the quality of life for those we care about by showing them affection in a variety of ways.

Love is expressed through hugs, pats, a protective arm around the shoulder, holding hands, and kisses. Or simply being there, smiling.

These can be important to a person who needs reassurance that someone still cares.

I will give hugs and asked to be hugged.

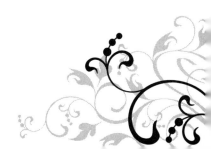

March 14 - Helplessness

Caregivers may feel the most helpless during the time when our loved-one may no longer recognize family and friends, or respond to the sound of our voice. Their mind seems to be gone, but the body remains.

As our loved-one becomes more and more ill, much of our distress lies in the fact that we can think of nothing that will help someone who is unresponsive.

I will continue to read to my loved-one and play soft music by the bedside.

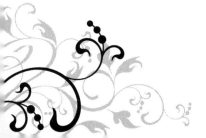

March 15 - Independence

It is very difficult for anyone to lose independence. Most of us prefer to make important decisions for ourselves. If a condition or disease is identified very early, it is possible to involve our loved-one in planning for the future.

Review the plan periodically with your loved-one. Allow them input for as long as they are able to communicate their wishes. This fosters the feeling of independence longer.

I will involve my loved-one in planning for their future.

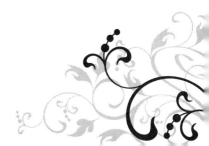

March 16 - Communication

As we get to know people, we also become familiar with their body language. By observing these non-verbal signals, we may discover that the moods they express are a consistent and accurate reflection of ideas and feelings that our loved-one/patient's are unable to put into words.

Caregivers can send as well as receive non-verbal messages. Our facial expressions, tone of voice, posture, firmness of our touch can make the difference between calming or scaring our loved-one.

I will remain calm, focused, and observant.

March 17 - Affirmation

Throughout the entire course of the illness it is very important to keep reaffirming the value of our loved-one/patient. We do this when we grieve together over the illness, and when we assure each other that we care.

We should let our loved-one know that he or she will not be deserted, and that he or she will continue to be an important part of the family.

I am loved and I love you.

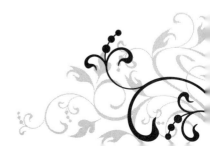

March 18 - Inner Self

Many of us are out of touch with our inner selves and the messages we send. We pay little conscious attention to our emotional responses. Beyond the recognition that we feel good or rotten we may be hard pressed to find words to express the things taking place inside.

Awareness of our feelings and emotions helps us to understand ourselves and can lead to healthier patterns of behavior.

I will listen to my inner voice.

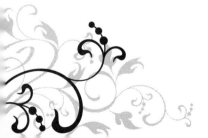

March 19 - Mental Pain

Buried pain is very much like a ticking time bomb. It ticks within, getting closer and closer to detonation, and can contribute to problems such as ulcers, heart disease, emotional disorders, and other aches and pains. It even contributes to alcohol abuse, drug abuse, overeating, and many other compulsive behaviors. It is a major factor in elder abuse.

I will face my own mental anguish daily.

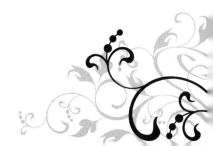

March 20 - Feelings

We must recognize that while all feelings are okay, all actions are not. We must take responsibility for all of our behavior, and recognize that each thing we do is a matter of conscious or unconscious choice. This differentiates us from our loved-one/patient, who may no longer be able to choose his/her behavior.

I will share my feelings with someone I trust.

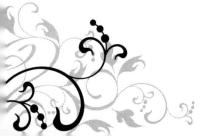

March 21 - Support

Caregiving for people who have Alzheimer's disease is a long, lonely, often misunderstood, and usually thankless responsibility. Because it is a prolonged experience, those who perform this function need a strong support system where thoughts, feelings, and concerns can be expressed.

I will join a support group.

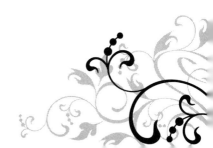

March 22 - Fear

It is a serious mistake to live in fear of something that may never happen. Fear of the future destroys present happiness. All we really have in life is the present moment.

The past cannot be changed. The future is unknown, but the present can and should be the very best we can make it.

Fear is a powerful stressor, and stress alone can confuse and distract us.

I am happy today. I will live in the moment.

March 23 - Guilt

It is unlikely that either we or the care-receiver planned to spend our middle or later years in a caregiving situation.

The changes in lifestyle, economic security, responsibilities, and relationships are accompanied by emotional responses.

These feelings are particularly troublesome because of the guilt which often accompanies them.

I.I.W.I.I. It is what it is and I will not feel guilty about it.

March 24 - Decisions

Smoldering feelings get in the way of decision making. Ignoring feelings does not make them go away. Feelings that are admitted and accepted can be placed in perspective and understood.

It may be inappropriate to express, or act out these feelings to the care-receiver, but recognition of them is important. In this way, we are freer to make the important decisions that we must make for our loved-one.

I will not let bad feelings get in the way of making good decisions.

March 25 - Coping

When feelings are not recognized or when they are denied and unresolved they can lead to conflict in relationships and to physical and emotional problems for the persons involved.

Caregivers can cope by accepting and acknowledging their feelings and by becoming aware of how the care-receiver is coping and what this is doing to the relationship.

We can also cope better when we develop skills in problem solving and decision making.

I reinforce what I learn in doing.

March 26 - Family

Family relations are not always warm, loving, cooperative situations. Often there is friction among family members as changes occur, and in some families the various members don't even like each other.

Role expectations are not clear, or people do not agree about what is expected of each other.

Conflicts can develop unless new roles and rules are defined and expectations are clarified within the individual and within the family.

I will do my best today.

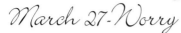

March 27 - Worry

Caregivers worry that their best efforts are not sufficient. We are fearful not only for the fate of our loved-one, but also for our own future.

We are concerned that onlookers (friends, healthcare professionals, family members) will fault us for our efforts.

We are grieved at the losses we see and those we anticipate.

I will allow myself to go through grief, but I am not worried that I am doing enough for my loved-one.

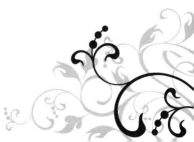

March 28 - Past History

Besides coping with the current physical and emotional changes in our loved-one, we may also be confronting problems that have surfaced from the past.

It is important to look at the expectations that people have for themselves and others.

I will let go of the past and live in the moment.

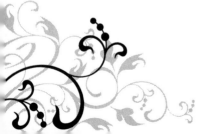

March 29 - Anger

Caring for older people can bring out anger related to their increasing dependency and demands of our time, energy, and money.

It is okay to be angry. However, it is what we do with our anger that is important. We must channel that anger into better care for our loved-one.

I will take a moment to get control of my emotions. I will act instead of react.

March 30 - Reminiscence

Reminiscence can be a valuable tool to be used by the caregiver of an elderly person. It can help the care-receiver to remember that his/her life has been of value.

It helps to place both positive and negative aspects of the past in perspective.

I will learn from our past experiences.

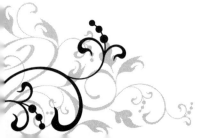

March 31 - Communication

Family members may have difficulty with communication because we take each other for granted or may have grown away from each other. We may have never really known much about the real feelings and values of each other.

We may have to develop new communication skills if we want to draw together for group decision making in support of our loved-one.

I will keep an open mind while I expand the lines of communication in my family.

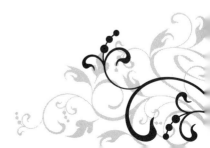

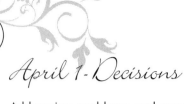

April 1 - Decisions

Addressing problems and needs associated with caregiving may involve more than one person. We need tools to help various family members to agree on what the problems are and to understand why certain decisions are being made.

Our emotional involvement may make decision making more difficult.

My best decisions reflect values and beliefs.

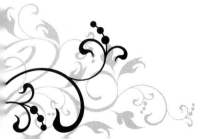

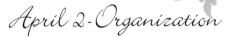

April 2 - Organization

Being a good advocate requires strong organizational skills. At the same time, we need to be firm but polite, assertive and persistent. These traits don't necessarily go hand in hand.

We need to share the workload and not be afraid to ask for assistance.

I will make a list of tasks and find out who can help.

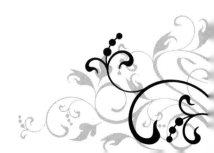

April 3 - Depression

For some caregivers, the emotional fallout from caring for a loved-one goes beyond stress and into the realm of depression. We might already be on alert for symptoms in our patient, but we should watch out for ourselves as well.

The burden of caregiving usually falls most heavily on one person. We have to take good care of ourselves.

I will schedule a check-up with my doctor.

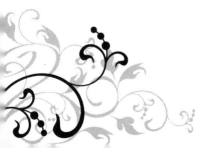

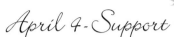

April 4 - Support

No one should feel isolated by their caregiving responsibilities.

Peer-to-peer support gives us a forum for relating our own daily struggles and learning how others cope with similar challenges.

We can reach out.

I will call another caregiver if I have questions or concerns.

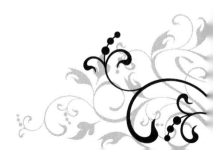

April 5 - Problems

We often get so bogged down in a situation that seems unmanageable or hopeless that we can't find a starting place for making decisions.

A good way to begin is by simply describing the situation. If other family members are involved, each should state the problem as he/she sees it.

Good ideas can be generated from listening to how others describe the problem situation.

With help, I will overcome all the problems of the day.

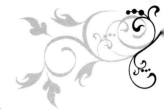

April 6 - Choice

The decision making process may lead to a decision not to act or not to try to change things.

This is may be a reasonable decision, and represents choosing to continue to do what is already being done.

Making a conscious choice to continue as is, or not to act, may be the perfect choice.

I am willing to begin where I am right now.

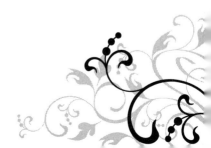

April 7 - Establish a Routine, Together

Both the caregiver and care-receiver will benefit from the time and effort spent choosing appropriate activities for the care-receiver. We all enjoy taking pride in what we accomplish.

Care-receivers need to experience this joy of accomplishment and are likely to experience a higher level of self-esteem if they successfully participate in activities.

I don't have to make all the decisions. But I am responsible for all outcomes.

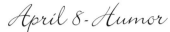

April 8 - Humor

A good sense of humor and a little laughter can work small miracles. Laughter stimulates the production of chemicals in the body which are natural anesthetics and relaxants.

As difficult as the prescription may seem, we will benefit by allowing humor into our lives. Watching silly TV programs, remembering old jokes, or even picking out ludicrous aspects of our situation can provide a needed break.

I will laugh out loud today.

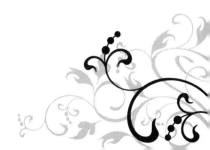

April 9 - Respite

We will find it easier to get through the day if we learn to take breaks.

These breaks, or respite periods, can include short relaxation exercises, short rests, reading periods, or physical exercise.

Breaks can also mean longer rest periods, such as a whole afternoon or a whole weekend away from the situation.

I will recharge my battery and eliminate any interferences.

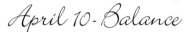

April 10 - Balance

Like most other people, we can benefit from a balance of activities in our lives. It is equally important for us to attend to our needs for socializing and emotional support, as it is to pay attention to our physical needs.

Going out to lunch, attending a class or attending a caregiver support group are all ways of taking a break. We should explore all options for respite services that can facilitate these outings.

I will call a friend to join me for lunch.

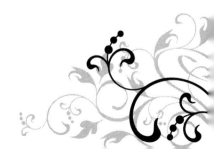

April 11 - Daily Management

By taking some time to think about our values and to decide which are the most important to us, will help simplify the management of our lives.

Each of us has different views about what is the most important. We should think about our expectations for our daily lives.

If we do not assert our rights, others may be managing us.

I know what is most important to me.

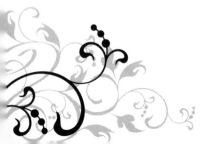

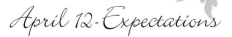

April 12 – Expectations

We should not expect that we will be able to solve every problem or control every situation. We must learn to accept what we cannot change or have no control over.

A focus on small problems, or small parts of a larger problem, is important. If we try constantly to solve the big problems, it puts extra stress on us.

We should try to simplify our lives as much as possible.

I will move beyond my old limitations.

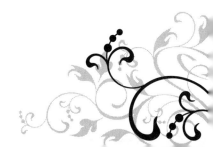

April 13 - Reflection

We must take one day at a time and enjoy each day. We must laugh at ourselves and the disturbing behaviors of our care-receiver. After each frustrating experience, we can take a moment to reflect on a past achievement. If we keep our mind on the pleasant aspects of life rather than worry about our problems, we will be able to maintain a more positive mental balance.

I relax and I let go.

April 14 - Attitude

The way we stand, sit or greet another person conveys subtle messages about our expectations and attitudes. Ideally our stance should convey assertive self-confidence and self-control and not passive or aggressive signals.

During interactions with family members we should be aware of the impression we are making.

I will show my family that our loved-one is in good hands.

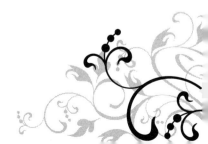

April 15 - Problem Solving

It sometimes helps to escape from a problem for a short time. Read a book, go to a movie, go for a walk, go for a drive somewhere.

It's not only therapeutic to escape our environment long enough to recover breath and balance, but to be prepared to come back and look at the problem when we are more composed.

My thinking is peaceful and calm.

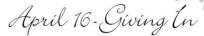

April 16 - Giving In

If we find ourselves getting into frequent quarrels and feeling defiant, remember that frustrated children behave the same way. We should stand our ground but do it calmly and remember that we could be wrong.

Even if we are sure we are right, it's sometimes easier to give in now and then.

I release the need to be right.

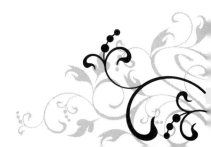

April 17 - Anger

While anger may give us a temporary sense of righteousness, or even power, it will probably leave us feeling foolish. If we have the urge to lash out, wait awhile. Take a deep breath and deliberately postpone lashing out until tomorrow.

When we replace that pent-up energy with something constructive, like walking or singing, our anger will subside.

Today I am strong and sound.

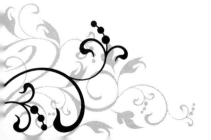

April 18 - Workload

For caregivers under tension, an ordinary workload may seem insurmountable. The tasks look so large that it may become painful to tackle any part.

Prioritize the tasks — do only a portion of it at a time. Do the biggest load first. Once the major task is done, the rest won't be so big any more.

I move forward with confidence and ease.

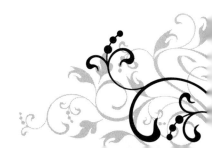

April 19 - Perfection

Sometimes we expect too much of ourselves. We strive for perfection in everything we do. The frustration of failure leaves us in a constant state of worry and anxiety.

We should give it our best. It will not be so bad if at the end, some tasks are not done exactly to perfection. We've given it our best — that's what counts.

I am a great caregiver.

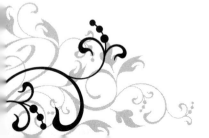

April 20 - Criticism

Expecting too much of others can lead to frustration and disappointment. We each have our own virtues, strengths, shortcomings, and values. Instead of being critical, we should search out the other's good points and help him/her to develop them.

If we only look at the negative side of others, we will likely look at ourselves negatively.

I will go easy on criticism.

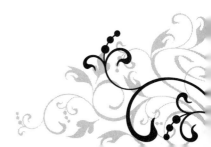

April 21 - Checklist

A checklist helps us maintain a fairly routine schedule without actually forgetting or ignoring areas that require less attention.

Keeping and maintaining schedules is an effective tool/aid in time management. This ensures that our chores are distributed throughout the day, week, or month, thereby making caregiving easier.

I am on schedule.

April 22 - Planning

Caregiving is difficult. Shouldering the work by ourselves is like being *"it"* in a game of tag. If we're lucky someone else will take their turn.

Lots of us remain *"it"* because no one else lives near or because they don't know how to get involved.

Anticipating the situations we are likely to encounter helps us to be better prepared.

I will share the care.

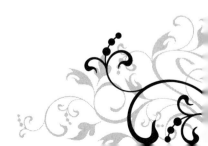

April 23 - Guilt

The bane of caregiving is that no matter how much we do, we always feel that we could have done more. Even worse is the guilt felt when angry words toward the care-receiver occasionally spring from our lips in the frustration of the moment.

Realize that we are doing the best we can with what's available. Our guilt will flow in and out along with other negative and positive feelings.

I forgive myself.

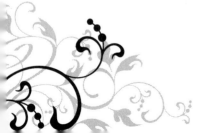

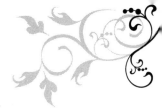

April 24 - Help

Don't let offers of help dry up. Every time someone offers, respond graciously with a specific task. Keep a list ready at all times, just for these occasions and add to the *"chore list"* whenever something needs doing.

Keeping uninvolved relatives in the loop about medications, treatments, and finances increases the likelihood of their involvement.

I am open to receiving help.

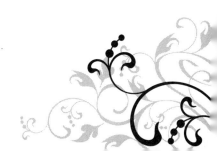

April 25 - Acceptance

It may be infuriating when others don't do their share, but ultimately we must accept that even though it makes sense to request their help, we can't force people to do anything they don't want to do.

In the long run, we're better off not spending time stewing over this, which only results in anger, bitterness, and family feuds.

If someone can't help, I move on to other people for support.

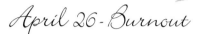

April 26 - Burnout

Caregiver burnout occurs when the amount of work that needs doing outstrips our time and energy.

Providing care, day in and day out, and getting very little in return also adds to caregiver stress.

When caregiving brings us nothing in return, not even appreciation, we should seek other sources of satisfaction, such as a support group or the warmth of a sympathetic friend.

I will confide in a friend today.

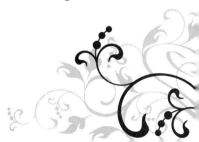

April 27 – Approval

Providing care in the hopes of getting a parent's approval or love may be a setup for disappointment. Whatever we choose to do, we must be clear about our expectations. Most deep-seated hurts and angers are not resolved as the end-of-life approaches.

We must accept our limitations — and those of our parents. The only approval we really need is our own.

Today I will let go of past hurts and anger.

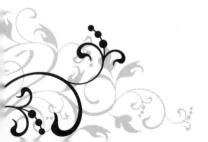

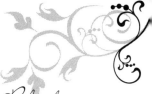

April 28 – Stress Relief

Stress relief strategies:
- Lighten up.
- Look for ways to save time and energy.
- Avoid isolation.
- Practice what we preach.
- Join a support group.
- Use relaxation techniques.
- Discover a new hobby.
- Rotate chores.
- Re-connect with an old friend.
- Compartmentalize tasks.
- Take advantage of respite care.

I adapt easily to change.

April 29 - Respite

Respite care is a simple remedy that prevents caregiver stress and burnout.

Respite works best when our time off is spent on activities that refuel, relax, and energize us. Regularly scheduled respite, whether for a few hours, a whole day or weekend, can boost our mental and physical well-being.

I will take a break today. For me!

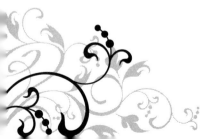

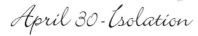

April 30 - Isolation

Caregivers need friends, too. Friends enhance our coping abilities with their listening, understanding, and advice.

Time spent with a friend produces a few good laughs and presents a distraction from our caregiving burdens.

Keep up phone contacts. Schedule regular coffee dates with friends

I have lots of friends.

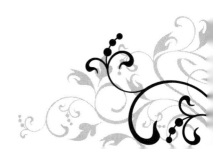

May 1 - Excitement

We should practice getting excited about the littlest things. Get excited about sunshine, inspired about rain or snow. If we are happy about our loved-one's smallest deeds, or in awe of a night full of stars, then our joyful attitude will carry over to any task about which we would like to be motivated. It may be surprising how much we will accomplish.

I am happy to smell the roses.

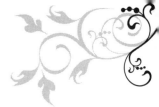

May 2 - Energy

We can get a quick energy boost by eating a piece of fruit (bananas, apples, pears, peaches, melons) or by having a glass of natural fruit juice or a high fiber energy bar.

Research has proven that *"nibbling"* at many points throughout the day is much more effective in delivering constant energy than three heavy meals a day.

I make meal choices that are beneficial for me.

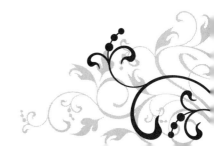

May 3 - Success

Embrace every success along the path.
At every step of the way, we should attribute any success to ourselves.

We can accept blame for failures too.
Consider these as the feedback we need to make positive adjustments in our strategy.

I love myself and trust the process.

May 4 - Knowledge

If we don't stay abreast of the knowledge brought about by modern technology, the trends in the marketplace, and the discoveries in healthcare, we will be left far behind.

By having the desire to stay familiar with these changes and being open-minded about them, our continued success is ensured.

I will learn something new today.

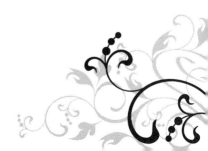

May 5 - Skills

Our attitude is enormously important; it enables us to accomplish many things. But without the right skills, we are limited in what we can do regardless of our attitude.

Without the skills to go with the right attitude, our success ceiling is limited. Remember, motivation precedes education. The best caregivers have the right attitude and the right skills.

I will seek to expand my skills today.

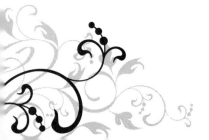

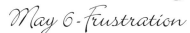

May 6 - Frustration

Most people are not trained to handle frustration, despite the fact that frustration is a daily event for most of us.

The inability to manage frustration has a greater impact on productivity and quality than intelligence and energy.

The solution to frustration starts with effective communication and honesty. And remember the old adage — honey catches more flies than vinegar.

I will be gentle, kind, and relaxed no matter the situation.

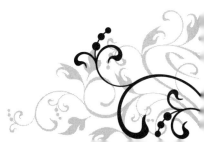

May 7 - Relationships

Our mental health and growth may be strongly influenced by a friend who listens quietly as we rave and rant about caregiving.

Maybe our pastor or counselor helps us stay mentally fit. Different types of relationships affect different levels of good mental health. The important thing to note is that relationships play a big role.

I will share my thoughts and feelings with a trusted advisor.

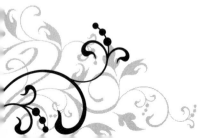

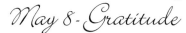

May 8 - Gratitude

The more we express gratitude for what we have, the more we have to express gratitude for.

We will never find a happy person who isn't a grateful person, so gratitude is a good place to start!

It also helps to magnify the important things and reduce the magnitude of problems that seem insurmountable.

I am thankful to be taking care of my loved-one/patient.

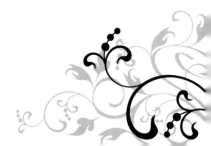

May 9 - Kindness

We must always treat our care-receiver/patient kindly, gently, and with respect and consideration. They will respond favorably.

On the other hand, if we are unkind and speak harshly, they are unable to perform at their best.

Kindness and consideration have many rewards, wherever we are and whatever we are doing.

I will be kind towards everyone.

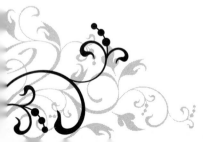

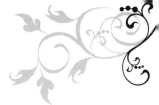

May 10 - Traits

What constitutes a good caregiver? The best caregivers share these traits:

- Conviction
- Commitment
- Hard Work
- Integrity
- Character
- Persistence
- Discipline
- Humor
- Connections
- Faith

Qualities shared by good caregivers are necessary to succeed in any area of life.

My good character is what powers me daily.

May 11 - Reality

Being a caregiver and loving what we do is a marvelous plus, but people make too much of it in one respect. Some people take it too far and interpret it to mean that we should love every aspect of caregiving. That is not realistic.

My work is a joy and a pleasure but I am realistic.

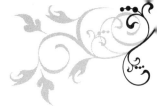

May 12 - Luck

Being at the right place at the right time may be better than being the smartest person in town.

However, most people appear at the right place at the right time not by luck but by hard work and determination. They get what appears to be a big break, but in truth, they worked hard to get where the big breaks come.

I will work harder today than yesterday.

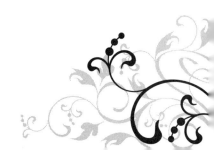

May 13 - Motivation

Motivated caregivers get more done. We move with a spring in our step, and we attack tasks with enthusiasm. We move quickly, deliberately, and with a concern for maintaining a can-do attitude along the way.

I'll go through my day with verve in my voice and a spring in my step.

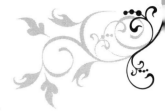

May 14 - Worry

If worry worked there would be no more poverty, war, famine, or tragedy in the world.

In reality, worry doesn't work at all. Even though laughter can't cure the world's ills, it sure can make us feel better. Our goal should be to laugh our way to good health.

I will not take myself so seriously today.

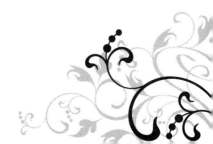

May 15 - Challenges

Every day we will have challenges and difficult situations to handle. There is a lot of help available to us if we look for it and ask for it.

The duties of a caregiver usually change and increase over a period of time. One of the most difficult aspects of the caregiver role is that the job continues 24/7/365. One way to get through each day is to set up a care plan and develop a routine.

With help, I will not be given more than I can handle today, or any day. I will ask for help.

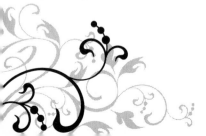

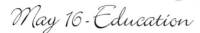

May 16 - Education

Educating our loved-ones/patients about their diagnosis and providing detailed, interactive information helps them to modify their behaviors.

Helping care-receivers take charge of their own care leads to an overall improvement in health.

Talking with our loved-ones about their diagnosis gives them comfort of knowing they are being looked after and helps reduce feelings of isolation, which can negatively affect their well-being.

I will learn more about my loved-one's condition and share it with them.

May 17 - Support

We (caregivers) need someone who listens and lets us talk about our feelings without being judgmental or giving unwanted advice.

Stressed caregivers often cannot provide good, safe care. Caregivers are at a higher risk for depression than the general population.

I will join a caregiver support group.

May 18 - Obstacles

One of the biggest caregiving obstacles we may face in helping a person who is seriously ill is the person himself/herself.

The idea that we can no longer take care of ourselves, or that we see that our loved-one cannot take care of themselves, brings up our deepest fears and our deepest wounds.

Before we can deal with our loved-one's denial, we may have to deal with our own.

Today I will be totally honest with myself.

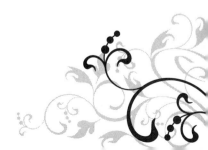

May 19 - Touch

When our loved-one is seriously ill, one of the things that often happens is that people stop touching them, just when they need a hug, a kiss, a hand, or a pat on the shoulder the most.

People in hospitals are rarely touched though research has shown that touch can enhance the healing process.

I will give out hugs every day.

May 20 - Involvement

It's very easy when we are caring for someone who is seriously ill over a long period of time to think of that person as identified with an illness. It's almost as if such people are the cancer.

Yet often people at the end of their lives have a great deal to give. So we shouldn't stop sharing our dreams, hopes, and our own problems.

I will be open today.

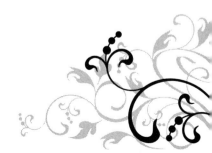

May 21 - Acknowledgment

Caregiving may be one of the most demanding things we will ever do.

We should give ourselves a treat after a tough assignment. Take a relaxing shower or a hot bath. Water seems to actually wash away the vibrations of illness, to renew us, and to restore us.

We must own our own goodness and acknowledge ourselves for doing whatever we can do.

I will not pretend my job is easy.

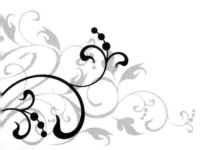

May 22 - Rewards

Being a caregiver can be joyous and enriching. It can be a time of increased sharing.

We can gain wisdom from care-receivers as they tell their stories and talk about what they learned in life.

We can gain satisfaction from knowing our care-receivers are receiving help.

I am a good listener.

May 23 - Encouragement

Caregivers are encouraged to attend medical appointments with our care-receivers. We can encourage them to be honest and explicit about symptoms at home. We can facilitate openness.

By attending appointments we will be better able to comply with medication directives and watch out for possible side effects addressed by physicians.

I contribute to my loved-one's well-being.

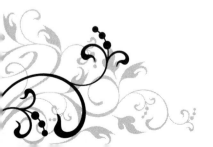

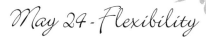

May 24 - Flexibility

We must resist the impulse to rush in and try to fix everything. We must respect our loved-one's needs to remain independent and allow them to do what they can do, even if their actions may not be up to *"normal"* standards.

We should focus on capacity (what the care-receiver can do) rather than incapacity (what the care-receiver can't do).

Each day gets easier.

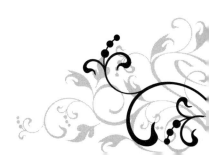

May 25 - Intervention

We must intervene gracefully and only when necessary. Caregivers must strive to make decisions with the care-receiver and not for the care-receiver.

We must respect the autonomy and sovereignty of care-receivers who, unless they are seriously mentally incapacitated, have the right to make decisions about their own lives.

I handle all my experiences with love and wisdom.

May 26 - Stress Management

Most caregivers experience enormous stress, which can wear on our health and lead to inadequate care for the patient/care-receiver.

We must mitigate our own stress, realize our limits, and set boundaries with our patients/care-receivers.

I will let go of stress today.

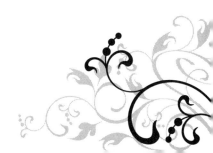

May 27 - Planning

We often spend 80 percent of our time on 20 percent of our chores. In order to maximize effectiveness, we need to establish processes that improve effectiveness.

We must establish workable plans, which include backups in the event of illness or emergency. Finding people to help with chores and other household duties is one thing we often forget to do.

I will review my plans.

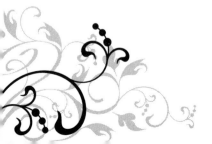

May 28 - Abuse

If unresolved family problems lurk beneath the surface, such as abuse, neglect, or denial of our emotional or financial support, a potentially dangerous situation exists because caregivers abused earlier in their lives assume positions of power over their abusers.

Even stable family relationships and positive perceptions of our care-receivers can become distorted as the demands of caregiving increase.

I release all blame.

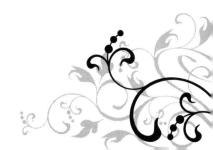

May 29 - Grief

Caregivers of loved-ones in clear decline experience anticipatory grief. The closer the bond between caregivers and care-receivers, the more stressing and fatiguing is the specter of death.

Proximity to the death process may be more stressful to family caregivers than to agency caregivers who, by training and experience, are better prepared for death.

I am supported by life.

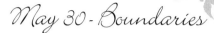

May 30 - Boundaries

Boundaries help us to define what we will and will not accept in our behavior and the behavior of care-receivers.

Boundaries assist in defining and respecting our *"no's"*.

Boundaries remind us of our responsibility to behave consciously.

Boundaries help us get priority needs met.

I will be aware of my and my loved-one's boundaries.

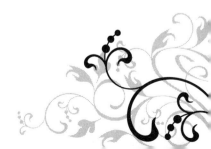

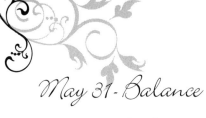

May 31 - Balance

We must actively take care of our own needs. We must:
- Pace ourselves.
- Delegate responsibilities to others, especially when stress levels are high.
- Vent feelings to friends or professionals.
- Attend classes, workshops to obtain new information and ways to cope with stress.
- Participate in leisure activities.
- Seek counsel.

I take care of myself the best I can.

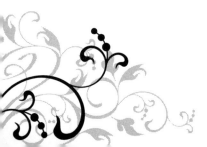

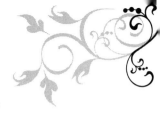

June 1- Options

Caregivers need options. We need information and assistance.

We need to know resources, both professional and volunteer, that are available in our local area.

Staying linked to our social networks, and even occupying multiple roles (worker, spouse, parent, etc.) is associated with better health, lower stress, higher self-esteem, and greater well-being.

There is something for me to learn in this role.

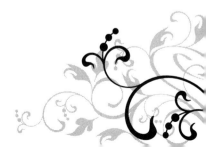

June 2 - Take a Break

Occasionally, we all feel frustration, guilt, fatigue, and isolation. Acknowledging this reality can be very healthy. Still, many of us have forgotten what it is like to take a break. In some instances, we have lost hope that anyone is willing or able to provide even occasional care to our loved-one/patient.

Respite care reduces the incidence of caregiver burnout and, over time can allow the care-receiver to live at home longer.

I will contact a family member or respite volunteer to provide some relief.

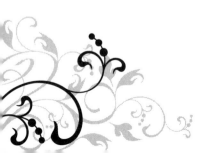

June 3 - Stress Mitigation

We must recognize what causes stress and establish a plan that will mitigate the stress. We must assess how we are doing on a daily basis by having a "How's it going?" assessment. We must ask ourselves:

- What's happening?
- How am I doing with what's happening?
- What do I need to change to make the situation better for me and the care-receiver?

I am balanced.

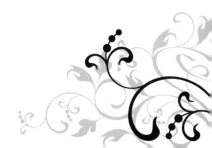

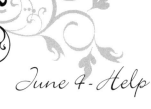

June 4 - Help

We must look for resources to help carry the load. Some resources to consider:
- Home health aides.
- Housekeeping services.
- Financial advisors.
- Insurance managers.
- Neighbors.
- Senior centers.
- Personal emergency response systems.
- Adult day care.
- Delivered meals.

I will accept help today.

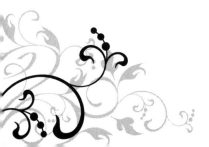

June 5 - Role Reversal

Role reversal is difficult. We are used to the care-receivers being the parents and in charge. Now we are. The role shift can lead to increasing caregiver frustration and/or guilt.

Care-receiver dependency is often not easy for the caregiver or the care-receiver.

I may be in charge, but we are all adults.

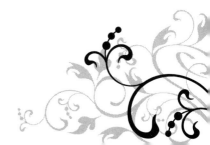

June 6 - Family Issues

Unresolved family issues often come to the surface in a caregiver/care-receiver relationship. The burden experienced by caregivers may be highly related to the number of social supports available from other family members.

Families either act as sources of support or catalysts for additional stress.

I am prepared for the possibility of burnout.

June 7 - Unequal Support

Sometimes life circumstances preclude some family members from giving direct caregiving support. However, those family members may provide financial support, calls to offer support to the caregiver and the care-receiver, or periodic respite care.

Although family members may not share equally in providing care to the loved-one, they need to be appreciated and involved in making decisions about caregiving.

I will share the care today.

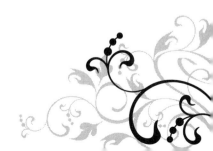

June 8 - Financial Stress

The financial stress of caregiving can compound the problems of the already burdened caregivers. The personal resources of both recipients and providers can be seriously drained by prolonged needs for care.

Decreased funding and increased utilization leads many agencies to direct their services toward primary pay clients, making these services even less available to those with low incomes.

I will keep my financial house in order.

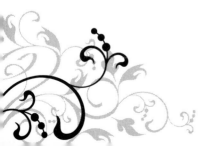

June 9 - Different Styles

Men and women define the caregiving role differently. Men tend to have a more instrumental focus, concentrating on tasks, goals, and problem solving, while women tend to be more person-oriented, concentrating on relationships, feelings, and the effects of their behavior on others.

Each approach has merit, but an attitude of positive concern for the care-receiver is the necessary requirement.

I will take good care of the care-receiver.

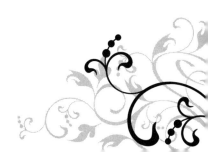

June 10 - Assistance

Caregivers tend to seek assistance only when the situation has reached an impossible extreme.

When services are brought into the care-receivers' homes, they are often marketed from a negative point of view. They emphasize *"relieving burdens"* rather than enhancing the caregiving relationship.

Caregiving is generally a burden AND a joy.

I will ask for more help before I need it.

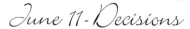

June 11 - Decisions

Shared decisions generally produce the best results. All participants will feel as if they own the outcome.

When planning on care we should ask these three questions:
- Who is most concerned?
- Who is most affected?
- Who has resources to offer?

Decision-making is a team effort.

I will take in all points of view from the caregiving team.

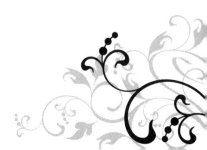

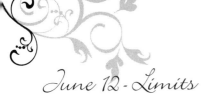

June 12 - Limits

It is vital that we keep ourselves in the equation of our own lives. Because caregiving is a difficult endeavor and often requires extraordinary commitment, energy, and time, we can easily ignore our own needs.

Over time, as we become absorbed in the care of our loved-one, we can cease to demonstrate concern for our own well-being.

I will establish and maintain loving limits.

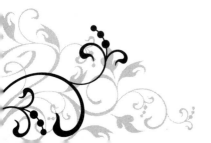

June 13 - Feelings

Caregivers cannot continue indefinitely when we are feeling strong negative emotions. We should ask ourselves where the emotions are coming from. We should be aware of the situations that elicit strong emotions in us.

Boundaries are often felt out rather than figured out!

I will listen to my feelings.

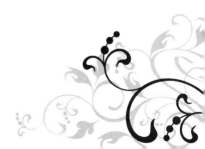

June 14 - Change

Give yourself permission to change the routine. If our guilt buttons are consistently being pushed and we cannot give ourselves this vital permission, we should seek professional counsel.

Caregivers who love their care-receivers and also love themselves will be healthier and more at peace as they strive to honor their caregiving roles.

I neither give or receive guilt.

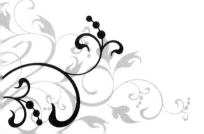

June 15 - Love

Our loved-ones want to be treated, and they have the need to be treated, as living human beings until the moment they die. Unknowingly, we *"protect them"* from the valuable opportunity to complete their lives. Too often we think of them as their diseases, by acting as if they are incapable of making their own decisions, by not acknowledging their opinions, by ignoring their desires, by withholding information from them, and by omitting them from conversations.

I will not rob my loved-one of their dignity.

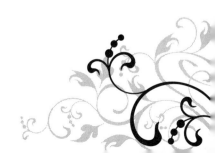

June 16 - Image

We each carry an image of ourselves in our heads. It's *"who we are"* in our minds. We see ourselves as something that transcends what we're going through.

The same thing is true for our care-receiver. They cling to that part of themselves that is changeless, that doesn't get lost and does not deteriorate with age or disease.

Their stories have not ended yet.

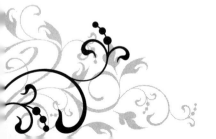

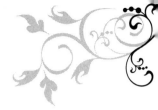

June 17 - Gifts

When our loved-ones first become sick, it is easy to see them as being whole people with a little bit of disease. As the illness progresses, our loved-one seems to become less of a person and more of a disease.

As caregivers, we have difficulty seeing the whole individual. Seeing beyond the illnesses is one of the most meaningful gifts we can give them.

Your spirit is changeless and I love looking into it.

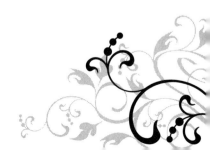

June 18 - Hope

Our lives are based on hope. We hope we won't lose control over our lives.

Hope and fear grip everyone who struggles with a life-challenging illness. If we take away hope, we are left with only fear.

Life is better for both caregivers and care-receivers when we live hopefully rather than hopelessly.

Hope should always be cultivated and never challenged.

I find hope every day, and in everything I do.

June 19 - Decisions

At any age, the choices we make are a reflection of our experiences, values, and desires.

Decision-making should be thoughtful and personal. We should attempt to include as many people as possible in the process, particularly if the decisions are made on behalf of other people.

I will make excellent decisions today.

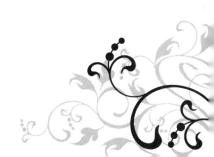

June 20 - Fear of Failure

Fear of failure plagues many caregivers. We must realistically take stock of our assets. Accepting them gives us the confidence we need to continue caregiving, and to meet our goals.

There is help available in support groups. All things become possible when we understand that we are not alone.

I am a good caregiver.

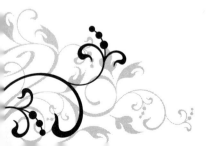

June 21 - Self-care

If we don't take care of ourselves, we can't possibly take care of another person. We have to remember to take some time for ourselves.

It helps if we get regular exercise. We also need enough sleep. Rest enables us to maintain the energy needed to provide care for ourselves and our loved-one.

It helps to talk with other people who may be in the same situation.

My health is important to me.

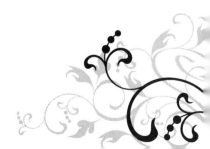

June 22 - Disagreements

As caregivers, we will likely encounter situations where we have to override the care-receiver's wishes to keep them safe and well. We should pick our battles carefully.

It is not possible to eliminate all disagreements and uncomfortable situations, but we can resolve conflicts and make our relationships run more smoothly.

I know when I don't have to have it my way.

June 23 - Encouragement

It is easy to complain when things aren't going right, especially when we are overwhelmed and exhausted. But instead of complaining when things go wrong, try praising our loved-one when things go right. Chances are our care-receiver wants to please us and will appreciate the encouragement.

I will see the good in every situation.

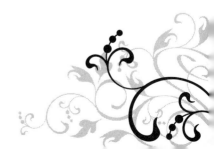

June 24 - Combatting Conflict

Even minor conflicts can escalate to epic proportions when we're faced with them day in and day out.

One key to being an effective caregiver, and minimizing head-butting, is to take a break now and then.

Take a break. Both you and your care-receiver will benefit from it.

I am willing to 'let my hair down' occasionally.

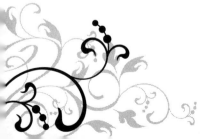

June 25 - Feelings

Negative feelings can make us feel uneasy and guilty, but it's important to understand that feelings of anger and resentment are natural and common.

Unless these feelings control us, and our behavior toward the care-receiver, they are not bad.

I will only have positive reactions irrespective of my feelings.

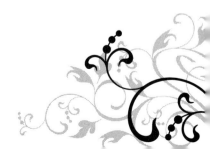

June 26 - Personality Patterns

Our basic personality patterns and traits don't change; and neither do those of the care-receiver. Our traits and patterns may even intensify over the years.

We should not fool ourselves that our loved-one will change from who they've always been, no matter what we think they should become.

And we should not fool ourselves about what we will become through the caregiving process.

I will stay open-minded to this experience.

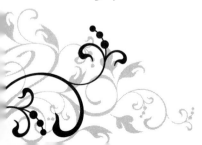

June 27 - Advice

Soliciting advice from our loved-one/elder is an effective way to open up a dialog. It makes them feel needed and appreciated.

Try these openers:
- Do you have any suggestions for me?
- What do you think about...?
- I want to get your opinion before I start...

And don't limit your questions to just caregiving. Your life issues can always use someone else's perspective.

I will seek advice and council from all my loved ones.

June 28 - Communication

Intelligence is not always what is needed the most during conversations with our loved-one — empathy is.

When we communicate love and concern, things go more smoothly. It requires time and patience.

We have to let our loved-one know that we care about their well-being.

I am gentle and caring.

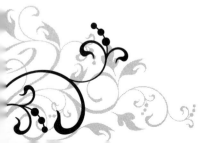

June 29 - Validation

Trying to talk anyone out of how he or she feels almost always creates distance and conflict between people.

We feel better when our point of view is understood. It is necessary to validate our loved-one's feelings. We don't have to agree with what is being said, but instead, simply that we understand what he or she is experiencing in the moment.

I am a good listener.

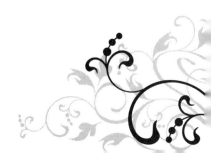

June 30 - Reality

Caregivers that find their role most rewarding don't live in a fantasy world about what's going on around them. We see the situation for what it is. We assess our responsibilities from where we stand, not from how we wish they could be.

We accept reality and roll with the punches. We do our best.

I accept responsibility for things as they are.

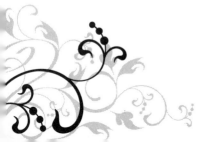

July 1 - Organization

There are things we can do to help keep the family organized. Designate a space for all caregiving papers, medical records, and legal records. An even better system is to store these records online at *www.MeAndMyCaregivers.com*.

As we plan our day and put our plan into action, resist the urge to do just one more thing, if it interferes with you taking care of yourself.

I am creating an organized life.

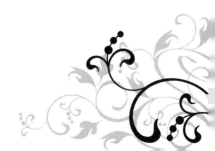

July 2 - Prayer

Caregivers can benefit from conversing with their Higher Power — out loud or silently.

Ask for help. Pray for the welfare of our loved-ones.

Offer thanks for the beauty and goodness in our lives.

I am grateful for my life.

July 3 - Happiness

Happy caregivers create and reinforce their moods. We can let ourselves be happy, but it takes work every day. We must have a purpose and a plan. We define what we want, and then use a strategy to get it. That creates happiness.

We can start by not taking ourselves so seriously. We can spare ourselves the clutter caused by bad feelings.

I am happy that I always do the best I can.

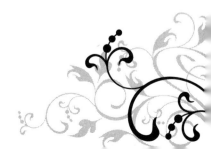

July 4 - Friendships

Because we care about others, we are cared for in return.

Even as busy caregivers we should take advantage of opportunities to expand our friendship base.

Close relationships are the most meaningful factors in happiness.

It helps to share our caregiving experiences with close friends.

I am blessed with many friends.

July 5 - Sleep

Caregivers who have a lot of anxiety let their thoughts bounce around from one subject to another as they try to go to sleep until, in short order they have created a whole catalog of problems.

We should limit ourselves to thinking about one subject as we lie down to sleep. When other thoughts start to intrude, we should guide ourselves back to that one subject.

Better sleepers are more satisfied with their lives than average sleepers.

I am a great sleeper and wake up rested.

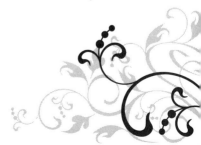

July 6 - Future

Our future evolves from the decisions we make, the priorities we develop, and the perspective we see things through.

We have been given life, and with it we have been given the opportunity to define it. Caregiving is just one part of our lives.

I will make my future what I want it to be.

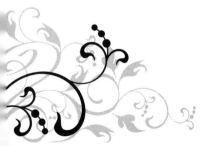

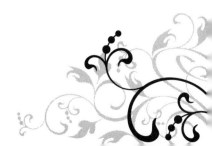

July 7 - Learning

Those of us who read books benefit from what we learn and the entertainment we receive. An added bonus is that we get to exercise our brains.

The more we read, the more skills we learn, the better caregivers we become.

I am learning more every day.

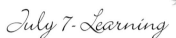

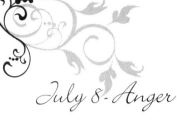

July 8 - Anger

There are steps we can take to help reduce the damage anger may have on our health.

- Write down our feelings. This is a wonderful way to vent.
- Exercise regularly.
- Take a relaxing bath.
- Take some time off, on a regular basis.
- Talk to a mental health counselor or medical doctor.

I am feeling warm and loving.

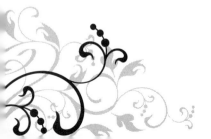

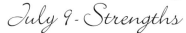

July 9 - Strengths

Caregivers face new and life-changing challenges every day. Conquering these problems often produces new coping methods and/or leaves us with more productive life-management strategies.

These new skills make us happier and more in control.

We should celebrate our strengths!

I am gaining new strengths.

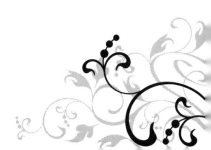

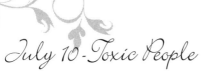

July 10 - Toxic People

Most caregivers struggle with issues from one or more toxic people (including family members).

Learning to say no, quickly and politely, is one of the keys to maintaining our own emotional and physical health.

We cannot afford to buy into their interference and manipulation, especially when they feel no responsibility to offer any concrete assistance.

I will say "no" quickly and politely.

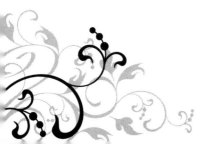

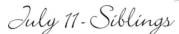

July 11 - Siblings

Sibling rivalry usually stems from long-term issues that can take years to alter. We can help ourselves by choosing our battles. We don't have to automatically respond to every comment, because not everything is important enough to argue about.

If we do respond negatively, we should step back and think about why we are angry. A calm, measured response gives us more control, and may help to diffuse the situation.

I am comfortable with my siblings.

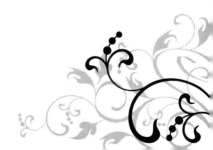

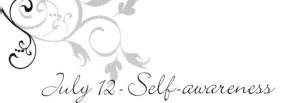

July 12 - Self-awareness

As caregivers, we should honestly believe that we deserve at least the same caring treatment that we provide for our loved-one.

We have the power to begin the process of self-awareness, insight, and progress toward taking care of ourselves.

Burnout and self-neglect are unacceptable.

I will take care of my needs as I take care of my loved-one's needs.

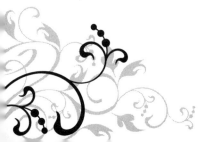

July 13 - Timing

Timing is everything. We should pay attention to our own natural body rhythms and schedule the most difficult caregiving tasks for our peak times of the day.

It is also important to realize that there will be times when someone or something will not receive immediate attention.

I am doing the best I can today.

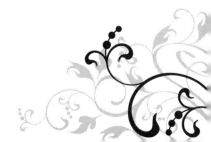

July 14 - Support

We cannot be successful without a support system. Caregiving, at best, is a series of wins and losses.

It is important to develop a network for assistance and support.

Practicing patience and delivering a kind word, peppered with *"please"* and *"thank you"*, will go a long way toward helping us generate the support we need to achieve our goals.

I am giving myself extra support today.

July 15 - Responsibilities

As our loved-ones need more assistance, we take on more responsibilities. As our duties increase, they take more of our time.

We must learn to manage our time.

Separating *"must do"* tasks and leaving the remaining ones for another time requires planning, practice and patience.

As I take on more responsibilities, I become a greater caregiver.

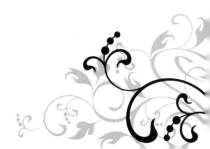

July 16 - Balance

Many caregivers are trying to balance workplace and caregiving issues.

For caregivers to remain emotionally healthy and productively employed, it is important to decrease workplace anxiety and interruptions, organize caregiving needs, and create solutions to relieve the pressures and fear that come from remote caregiving duties from the workplace.

I am creating solutions to caregiving problems.

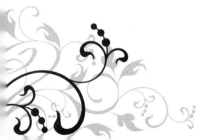

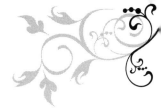

July 17 - Goals

Completing any goal we set for ourselves improves our confidence and satisfaction.

We need to be able to measure our caregiving progress, to know that things are improving. We can't accomplish an abstract goal, because we will never know if we are finished or not.

Making a list of things to accomplish each day will help keep us focused.

I am great at setting goals.

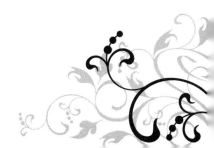

July 18 - Exercise Regularly

Caregivers who exercise, whether that involves an intense workout or just a regular walk, feel healthier, feel better about themselves and their care-receivers, and enjoy life more.

Regular physical activity can help to reduce stress and avoid caregiver burnout.

I am feeling warm and healthy about myself.

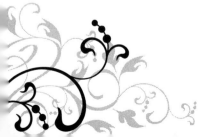

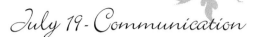

July 19 - Communication

Teeny, tiny things — the tone of our voice, the exact words we use as we go through otherwise ordinary caregiving events — communicate volumes.

Facial expressions and reactions are important to our communication.

Little things can have big meanings.

I am a great communicator.

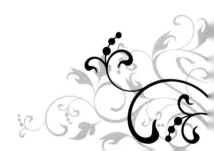

July 20 - Asking for Help

Many times, we want and need help but don't ask. Asking for help is not a sign of weakness; it takes courage to ask for help.

Once we admit needing help, we may find that it comes from the most unexpected sources.

We must remain open to receiving help even from unlikely sources.

I am open to receiving help.

July 21 - Self-care

To be a caregiver, we need to take care of ourselves. We need enough rest and time away from the care-receiver.

We need friends to enjoy, and to share our problems with.

We may find that we need additional help to cope with our feelings of discouragement or to sort out the disagreements in the family.

Finding ways to meet our own needs often takes effort and ingenuity.

I lovingly take care of my mind and body.

July 22 - Frustration

Anger and frustration are normal responses to caring for a person whose behavior is difficult.

However, if our anger spills over into other relationships or if we take our anger out on the care-receiver, it becomes our duty to manage our frustrations so that they do not drive people away from us or make the care-receiver's behavior worse.

I am at peace. I release my frustrations.

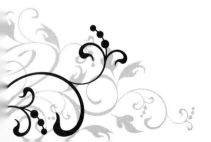

July 23 - Finances

Providing care for the person with a chronic illness can be costly. It is important to assess both available financial resources and potentially increasing costs of care, and make plans for the care-receiver's financial future.

Many factors must be considered in assessing our financial future, including the nature of the illness of the care-receiver, and our individual expectations.

I will make a sound financial plan for my loved-one.

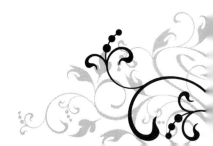

July 24 - Parents

We don't have to like our parents, but it feels better if we love them. After all, they gave us life — the greatest gift of all.

Whatever else they did or didn't do, if not for them, we wouldn't be here. They deserve a big thank you.

I see love and tenderness.

July 25 - Breathing

Caring for someone who is chronically ill, or who requires constant attention, is an extremely demanding job. We can give ourselves a mini-recharge by focusing on taking slow deep breaths, inhaling through the nose, and then exhaling gently and completely through the mouth.

A good dose of oxygen to the brain will produce noticeable effects immediately.

I nourish myself. My mind is at peace.

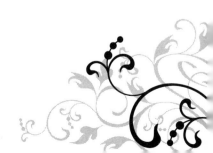

July 26 - Anger

We can slow down or stop the flow of anger and frustration by simply counting to ten before we speak.

When we slow things down and focus on counting, we can engage our rational brain and regain control. This can help keep our emotions from running amuck.

I will not let anger control me.

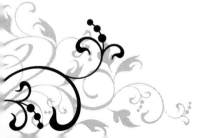

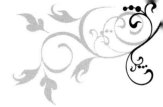

July 27 - Trust

Trust is built over time by open communication, willingness to share, consistency in words, actions, and behavior.

To build trust we must use our self-awareness and self-management skills.

Cultivating a relationship with the care-receiver, and building trust, may take time.

I am trustworthy in all I do.

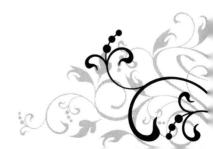

July 28 - Decisions

It helps when we take the time to explain why we made a decision, rather than just making the decision and moving on.

If we can ask for ideas and input ahead of time, it's even better. Then acknowledge how the decision will affect everyone.

Transparency and openness make people feel like they are trusted and respected.

I am a great decision maker.

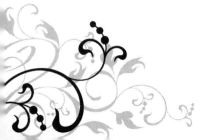

July 29 - Release

Crying, like laughing, is a wonderful natural release. We feel good after a cry or laugh.

Tears are natural to healing and enjoyment. We are often moved to tears from intense feelings of gratitude, awe, or compassion.

We should allow ourselves to be moved by our lives, and cry a little bit.

I release with joy.

July 30 - Forgiveness

To forgive another is being in favor of forgiving yourself.

Forgiveness is powerful and effective. You may not be able to forgive every day, but you should forgive whenever you are presented the opportunity.

I release and dissolve the past.

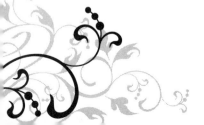

July 31 - Support

Joining a support group is an extremely valuable coping strategy, especially for the isolated caregiver.

The group experience can provide education, emotional sharing, resource information, and problem solving techniques.

We can develop a social support system that offers companionship and active help in crisis situations.

I reach out safely.

August 1 - Death

If our loved-one is near death, he/she needs to be shown unconditional love, free of our expectations and judgments.

Acceptance means that we caregivers impose no reservations, no conditions, no evaluations, and no judgments about our care-receiver's feelings.

It is important that we show a total, positive regard for them as people of value, whether we agree with their attitudes and decisions.

I hold no malice in my heart. All is well.

August 2 - Assessments

When working with a care-receiver, if we can assess for strengths rather than weaknesses, the person being assessed will receive a positive and empowering message: *"You do have some control. You have the capacity to solve your own problems."*

Established strengths can be reinforced every day.

I will look for the I cans, not the I can'ts.

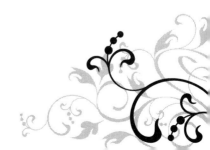

August 3 - Help

When we direct our conversations toward the good aspects of our lives rather than dwelling on the negatives, we can allow people to fuel their own positive energy.

We enable our care-receivers to have a sense of control when we direct our conversations in a more positive manner. We need to put more effort into looking for strengths.

I support my loved-one in healthy ways.

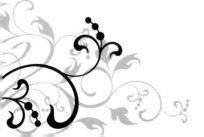

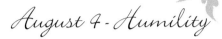

August 4 - Humility

We caregivers need to be humble in life so that we can facilitate choices and control for those in our care.

To do this, we must first recognize our own shortcomings and our own dependence on others.

We must develop within ourselves, a greater degree of humility through our patience, compassion, courage, fidelity, self-control, gentleness, love, truthfulness, sincerity, sense of humor, and friendship.

I am humble and stand in truth.

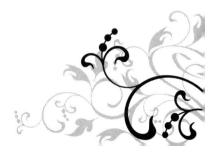

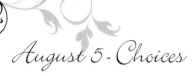

August 5 - Choices

We should promote choices whenever possible. The more choices, the better.

The chance to make choices is important to a sense of purpose because it enables the care-receiver to be an active participant in determining his/her fate.

Participation is a prerequisite to believing that his/her actions can make a positive difference in his/her life.

I rejoice in my choices.

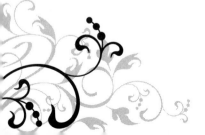

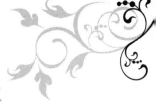

August 6 - Grief

When we show our grief openly we are also showing our love openly. The longer we postpone facing death, the greater hold our fears have on us and the care-receiver.

Knowing is less painful than not knowing. The quality of our lives is diminished when the truth is not recognized or spoken.

I am able to move forward with ease.

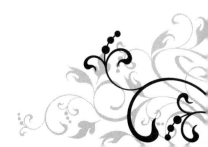

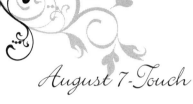

August 7 – Touch

Many caregivers overlook older people's desire for touch. The need for touch increases with age and during times of stress and isolation.

We would do well to recognize touch as an integral part of our caregiving skills.

We must also respect the care-receiver's choice about when touch is inappropriate — when it may be the wrong time, the wrong amount, or from the wrong person.

I feel love in every touch.

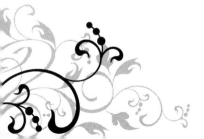

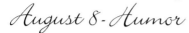

August 8 - Humor

Humor is an essential reminder of the joys of being a human being.

A good laugh can restore perspective. Laughter allows us to step back for a moment and regroup.

Appropriate humor depends on the right person, right time, and right dose.

The opportunity to laugh can benefit both the caregiver and the care-receiver.

I allow humor and joy to flow through me.

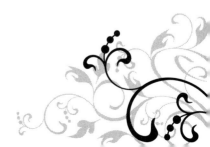

August 9 - Stress

When caregivers are under stress, we are not as able to meet the urgent needs of the people in our care.

Try these stress-reduction activities throughout the day:
- Clap your hands fifteen times.
- Make five different silly faces.
- Raise your eyebrows 25 times.
- Sing a song.
- Repeat.

I release negative thoughts from my mind and body.

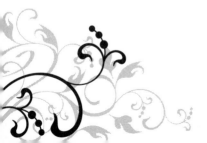

August 10 - Benefits

While there are many benefits associated with being a caregiver, it takes planning, support, and patience to excel.

Remember, we are not alone.

Many others are facing the same challenges. There are new techniques and services being developed and improved to help make our job easier.

To make our caregiving experiences rewarding, we must stay apprised of the newest, essential caregiving information.

I will improve my skills as a caregiver.

August 11 - Care Plan

Our care plan must be flexible enough to meet the continually changing needs of the person being cared for.

It's a good idea to consult with the other members of the caregiving team — such as doctors, nurses, pharmacists, family members, neighbors, community helpers — to develop the best plan to deal with our unique situation. Our plan should be reviewed and updated on a regular basis.

I am organized and accept new challenges.

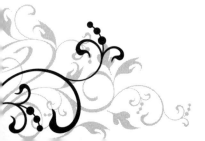

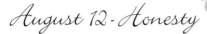

August 12 - Honesty

We must be honest with ourselves about what we can and cannot do. When we start to feel that the responsibility is overwhelming, we must ask others for help.

To be better prepared to accept offers of help, it is a good idea to keep a list of all the things that need to be done.

Trying to do it all ourselves is counterproductive and may even be dangerous. We should get in to the habit of asking for help as soon as we need it.

I know when to say when.

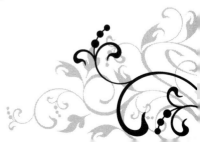

August 13 - Burnout

To help prevent burnout, we must have a dependable support system in place consisting of people we can talk to or visit on a regular basis to express our feelings and concerns.

Many caregivers are relieved just by having someone to talk to.

If nothing is done to relieve it or reverse it, burnout can lead to depression. While caregiving is not always a personal choice, it is a generous act.

I am not bulletproof. I will take care of myself.

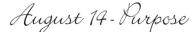

August 14 - Purpose

We are all connected. We are all affected by the decisions and even the existence of those around us.

Our lives have purpose and meaning. It's important to share with others how important they are to us.

We don't win at relationships, we win by having relationships.

I choose to be a winner.

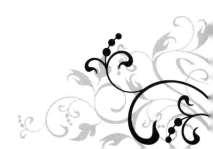

August 15 - Help

Caregiving problems can appear to be unsolvable. We are social creatures who need to discuss our problems with others, whether it be those who know us best or other caregivers who have faced the same problems we have.

When we are alone, problems get worse. By sharing, we can gain perspective and find solutions. We should not face our problems alone. Ask for help.

I will muster all of my resources so I can give better care.

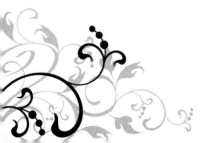

August 16 - Attitude

Our caregiving journey toward success will flow more smoothly if we have the right attitude.

A can-do outlook helps us to become solution-finders and to look for the good instead of the bad in everything.

It's important to have the right attitude toward our family, friends, and caregiving associates. An attitude of acceptance, forgiveness, love, kindness, respect, and consideration goes a long way.

I am happy and show it in everything I do.

August 17 - Knowledge

If we don't stay abreast of the caregiving knowledge brought about by modern technology, the trends in the marketplace, and the discoveries in the field of health improvement, we will be left behind, or at best, will experience only a portion of the progress that we are capable of experiencing.

We owe it to ourselves and to our loved-ones to learn as much as possible.

I learn new things every day that enrich my life.

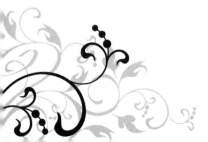

August 18 - Integrity

Caregivers with integrity do the right thing, when no one else is watching. When we have integrity, we have nothing to fear because we have nothing to hide. In doing the right thing for the right reason, we experience no guilt and no fear.

I approve of myself and all that I do.

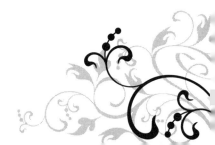

August 19 - Frustration

The inability to manage frustration has a greater impact on productivity than intelligence and energy.

We can turn our frustration into a positive by doing something constructive instead of destructive.

Good communication reduces our frustration and makes it easier to build and maintain a better relationship with our care-receiver.

I calm my thoughts and feel at peace.

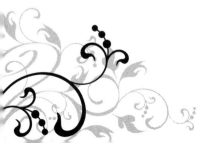

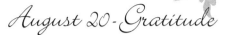

August 20 - Gratitude

The more we express gratitude for what we have, the more we have to express gratitude for. We will never find a happy caregiver who isn't a grateful person, so gratitude is a great place to start in order to be a happy caregiver.

Grateful caregivers are a joy to be around.

I appreciate every situation that comes my way.

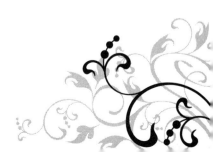

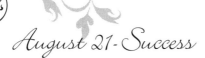

August 21 – Success

The hallmarks of success in caregiving are the same qualities needed in all areas of life. These include:

- Conviction
- Commitment
- Hard work
- Integrity
- Character
- Consistency
- Persistence
- Discipline
- Humor
- Luck
- Faith
- Passion
- Connections

I am a success in all I do.

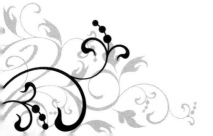

August 22 - Communication

Words can have a positive impact on our caregiving experience.

Kind, inspiring words with a helpful intent and a gentle tone of voice, help us build better relationships.

The most important words we can say to our loved-one is *"I love you."* The second most important words we can say are *"I made a mistake. Please forgive me."*

Other important words are *"please"*, *"thank you"* and *"you're welcome"*.

Words can improve our lives.

I am open and easy to talk to.

August 23 - Support

Caregivers must have a system of support. We require all kinds of support: equipment support, skills support, support in family situations, support in providing thorough care.

I am open to more help.

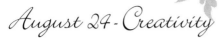

August 24 - Creativity

Another vital quality of an effective caregiver is creativity. Often we limit creativity to the arts, but creativity can be manifested in many ways.

Creativity can be demonstrated in any activity in the way things are done.

The crux of all creativity is the courage to change. Conversely, change requires creativity.

I embrace change.

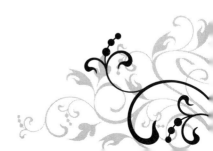

August 25 - Self-Talk

One of the ways to maintain a positive approach to caregiving is to *"speak it"*. When we speak, it reflects the state of our mind.

We can talk ourselves into attitudes, fears and sickness. We can talk ourselves out of these things, too.

To change our attitude we must change our self-talk. Our minds and bodies react towards our thoughts.

I am aware of the goodness in my thoughts.

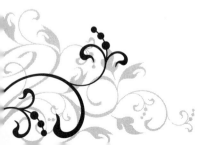

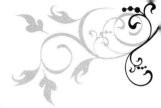

August 26 - Tact

Tact is all about thoughtfulness towards others and is a combination of interest, sincerity and caring.

We need to use care and sensitivity when communicating with the care-receiver.

Ill-advised or poorly expressed sentiments never assist anything but failure.

I am polite and compassionate.

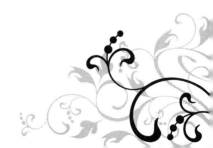

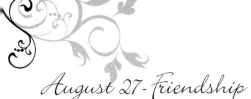

August 27 - Friendship

Friendship is a key factor for any caregiver. We will never be a good caregiver without first learning how to build simple human relationships.

The friends we surround ourselves with will be the friends who influence us in our thinking and decisions.

We must never take friends and friendship for granted, but rather should work hard on these relationships.

I am wealthy with good friends.

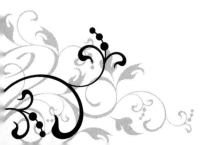

August 28 - Recreation

Never get too busy caregiving to play. Have fun!

Our period of recreation should be a time when we can purposefully get our mind off of caregiving, and be with ourselves, our family and our friends.

We need time to think about something other than our work or our problems.

Having specific intentions for relaxation time will assist us in maximizing our personal and professional potential.

It's time to play!

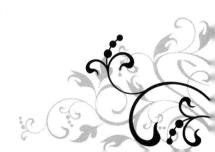

August 29 - Intentions

By designing a caregiving blueprint for our lives, we accept responsibility for how good we can become.

We begin by planning for our day, every day! We create tomorrow the night before. When we get up in the morning we know what we are going to do. Things get done when we plan them.

Set priorities on each item: must do, should do, and could do.

My prior planning prevents poor performance.

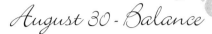

August 30 - Balance

When we set caregiving goals, we begin to create balance. To have balance in our lives must be a high priority.

Balance keeps us well rounded. It keeps us from going overboard in one area.

Regardless of what we choose today, we must do the best we can do.

I see clearly what my life balances around.

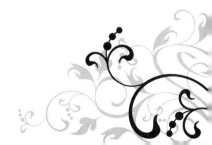

August 31 - Sharing

We are called to share our lives with others. Our contribution is like a candle. The candle does not lose any of its power by lighting another candle.

In fact, as long as a candle burns, there is no limit to the number of other candles it can light.

A simple word or gesture can serve to bring inspiration or healing to someone else's life. Our responsibility is to keep our own light shining brightly.

I am doing what I love.

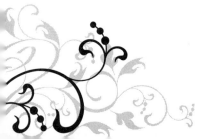

September 1 - Pressure

Everyone has certain mental pressure points. The trick is to focus on ours and develop strategies to deal with them.

We must prepare ourselves for pressure. We shouldn't be surprised when pressure brings out extraordinary results. When we embrace pressure and make it work for us, it can be a healthy climate in which we can flourish.

I relish all challenges.

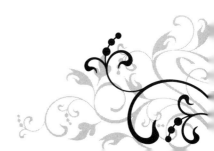

September 2 - Creativity

Being creative about caregiving solutions gives us additional motivation to face what we do every day.

Flexibility and adaptability are habits that can be cultivated and critical to maintaining the enthusiasm we need for persistence.

We have to look at each day as a new opportunity to change our lives as we take care of our loved-one.

Each moment is unique and an opportunity for me to grow.

September 3 - Adversity

Adversity happens to all of us, and it happens all the time — especially while caregiving.

Some form of major adversity is either going to be there or else it's going to be lying in wait. To ignore it is to succumb to the ultimate self-delusion.

Adversity requires that we step back and evaluate our role in the situation and determine the lessons we can take away.

I am clearing out old confusion and doubt.

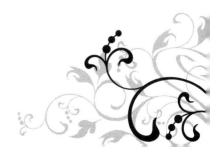

September 4 - Habits

The only way we can systematically acquire good habits is by staying organized.

We start off each caregiving day knowing there is a purpose in everything we do. We control and shape our day with our actions.

If we are not organized we set ourselves up to be unfocused, and quite possibly to fail.

My actions today are my habits of tomorrow.

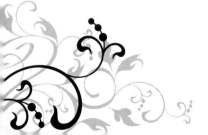

September 5 - Communication

We must communicate both our needs and goals to the care-receiver so that they can benefit from this knowledge. People want to know why they are being asked to do things. They want to be a part of the process.

Our goal is to communicate better, not to try to win every discussion or treat every conversation as if it's a contest with a winner and a loser.

Today I am not afraid of silence.

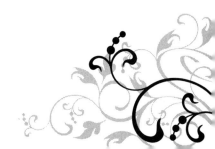

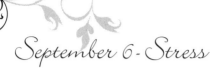

September 6 - Stress

As we struggle with caregiving challenges, we must differentiate between stress and pressure.

Stress is the enemy. It robs us of our focus and inhibits our performance.

Pressure is only a negative if we allow it to be.

It focuses our efforts on the important goals and concentrates our power where it counts.

I celebrate myself today.

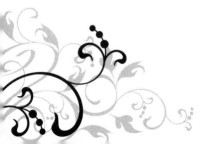

September 7 - Attitude

We can control our moods. A mood is simply a reflection of our attitude and we can certainly change our attitude.

We can look honestly at the reality of the situation and see the positive in it, while enhancing the quality of life.

We can program ourselves to be positive. Being positive is a disciplined attitude.

Being positive is contagious. When we are positive, our care-receivers are more positive.

I deserve wonderful things to happen.

September 8 - Relationships

Caregiving requires a relationship, more than a formula. It's daily living that really matters.

It is easy to slip into the mode of just completing today's tasks. But those tasks exist to take care of someone. That someone is the key.

And that someone can bring a lifetime of experiences to you if you take the time to build on the relationship you have with them.

Nothing can stop me from growing today.

September 9 - Perfection

Do not confuse striving for excellence with wanting to be perfect.

Striving for excellence is doing our best in the face of having no guarantees of success. But demanding perfection of ourselves will only become fuel for low self-esteem.

There will always be times when our best is not good enough to overcome the prevailing conditions.

Peace and relaxation flow through me.

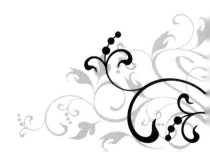

September 10 - Conflict

Conflict is invariably part of the caregiving experience. When we internalize a conflict and make it personal, we let an isolated situation/failure become a hallmark of our own inadequacy.

Rather than internalize a conflict, it is better to take the experience and apply it as a point of reference for all future experiences. Thus, a failure in one area does not automatically mean a failure in every thing we do.

Today I am establishing rapport with everyone.

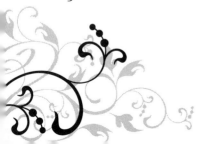

September 11 - Consistency

Decisions are not decisions if they are not backed by action and consistency. Without these two factors, belief and dreams are merely fantasies, knowledge and education are fruitless, and outside help goes unheeded.

The power of caregiving is in the doing! We must be committed to action.

I have a purpose today.

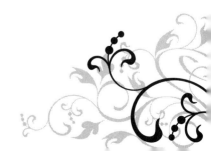

September 12 - Health

Our needs and desires, our emotions and thoughts, equally influence our health.

Our relationship with ourselves is delicate and needs nourishing and balance.

We all know what we need to do, but we have excuses, reasons, expectations, and blind spots.

Now is the time to address our needs.

I experience life as a joyful dance.

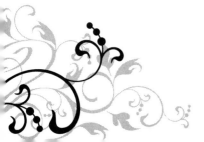

September 13 - Stress

Stress is a fact of life, especially for a caregiver. Let it be a friend in our health, and not a factor in our disease.

Stress can motivate our behavior, and even improve our performance. We control stress by using it as an opportunity, a challenge, and a priority.

Stress has no control over us, unless we empower it.

I will channel my stress for the positive.

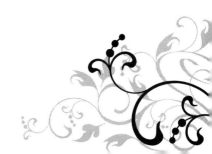

September 14 - Limitations

We can only do so much in one day. Let the rest go. Work smarter, work better, then stop.

We must spend time with our family and friends. Play hard and rest well.

Leave the stress behind — don't carry it from one day to the next.

When we are living in the moment, worry has no home.

I accept myself and am grateful that I can grow from where I am.

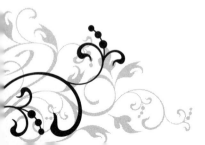

September 15 - Beliefs

Life is not about being perfect, but it is about being purposeful. We need a philosophy, a belief system, a game plan for our daily lives.

Our actions reflect our beliefs and help us get what we want. This is our test.

We must know ourselves and live by our principles.

I am open to positive changes.

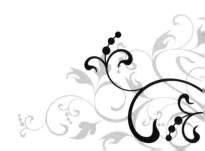

September 16 - Encouragement

Everyone needs and responds to encouragement. Encouragement is oxygen to the soul.

When we say something uplifting in the first sixty seconds of a conversation, it sets a positive tone for everything else.

Every successful caregiver knows that the best way to bring out the best in others, is by encouragement.

I reach out and see the best in others.

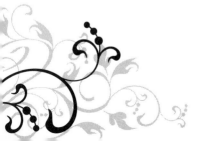

September 17 - Listening

Being a good listener does not come naturally to most people. It is a learned skill that comes with practice.

A good caregiver needs to learn active, reflective, effective and sensitive listening skills.

Listening, interspersed with questions, can be a helpful approach towards working with your care-receiver.

I am teachable and a good listener.

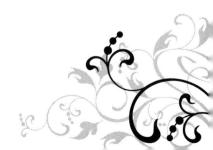

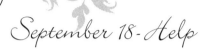

September 18 - Help

Ask for help. Don't wait for others to offer.

Talk with your family and members of the care team on a regular basis about the many responsibilities involved. Ask each person to commit to help.

For most caregivers, there are never enough hours in the day. Make a list of tasks others can do. Learn to let go. It's unrealistic to think we can do everything ourselves.

I am open to letting others help.

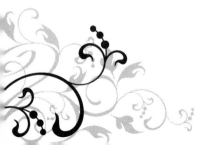

September 19 - Change

Change is a natural process of life. We can choose to make positive changes in ourselves, even while caregiving, that will improve our quality of life.

When we are conscious about our choices (rather than simply reacting to circumstances) and following through with them, we are making a commitment to ourselves.

Allow time to change and focus on the process.

I change my life when I change my thinking.

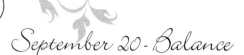

September 20 - Balance

It is important to plan to do something we love every day.

We can start by detaching ourselves slightly from our caregiving environment. We can use this as a technique for becoming more objective about our role as a caregiver.

When we are more objective observers, we are more likely to find ways to improve our balance.

I am centered.

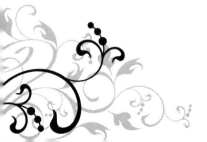

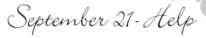

September 21 - Help

So often, we want and need help but don't ask.

Asking for help is not a sign of weakness; it takes courage to ask for help.

After we ask for help we must let others do the helping. It does no good to micromanage the person who is trying to relieve our burdens.

I am being supported by powerful energy.

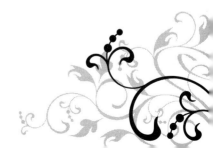

September 22 - Transformation

Impossible tasks remain impossible if we don't attack them and break them down into the possible.

That means taking what we have to work with and using it to our best advantage.

With hard work and determination we can persevere. We should remember that other caregivers have overcome similar challenges.

I am discovering who I really am. I am worthy.

September 23 - Distractions

We know that in caregiving issues or personal conflicts we can get tied up by *"overthinking"* a problem. We spend too much time *"what-if-ing"* instead of simply tackling the task at hand.

At some point the best we can do for ourselves is to jump right in and do it.

Oftentimes we have to put distracting thoughts out of mind.

I am focused. I can take another positive step forward.

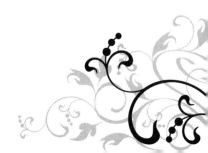

September 24 - Attitude

Attitude is key. It influences not only what we aspire to but how quickly we can get there without alienating our loved-ones or making ourselves crazy.

A positive attitude will take us a long way if it is coupled with being organized and believing in ourselves while we are doing our tasks.

Positive attitude produces confidence.

I choose to be positive today.

September 25 - Visualization

Visualization and positive self-talk are closely related. If we imagine ourselves as strong, compassionate, and capable, we can also tell ourselves the same things.

Along with our image we can create words that can be repeated as a mantra to enhance our performance.

We see it, say it, and become it.

I see the strength within myself.

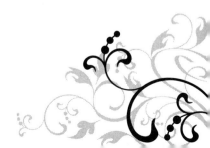

September 26 - Effectiveness

Because much of caregiving success is attributed to mental fitness skills, it's important that every caregiver, of every level, find the way to best prepare his or her mind as well as body to perform.

The method itself doesn't really matter – its effectiveness does.

I trust that I'm where I need to be today.

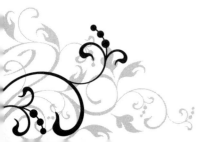

September 27 - Doubt

If we are constantly doubting what we can do, we will soon find that we won't be able to do it. Our mind can convince us one way or the other so it's better to get our mind working with us, not against us.

Belief in ourselves can come long before any technical prowess.

Simply believing that we are great caregivers takes us closer to meeting our goals.

I am letting go of negative thoughts.

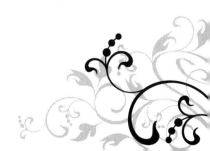

September 28 - Confidence

We are more apt to lose confidence when we get discouraged by lack of results.

It takes a special caregiver to stay focused and positive even in the most challenging of circumstances.

We can work on this skill. We can practice affirming our performances and praising ourselves for our motivation.

I know I can do it!

September 29 - Exercise

Exercising can help us to burn off steam. Instead of screaming, yelling, or throwing things, getting physical, positively, can be a very constructive way to vent our anger or frustration.

Exercise is great for getting our bodies toned and our hearts healthy, and our minds clear. Exercise can lift our spirits.

I am being renewed and refreshed by exercise.

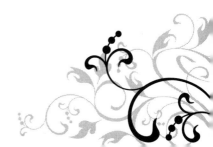

September 30 - Motivation

By demanding more from ourselves on a regular basis, we'll get more out of ourselves when we really need it.

We all have days when we just don't seem to have the energy or the interest in working at peak effort. These are the times to reach inside ourselves and try to find that extra umph that will motivate us to work harder.

Average is not good enough for me.

October 1 - Comfort Zone

Caregiving takes us out of our comfort zone. We overcome fear, guilt, hurt feelings, and anger as our comfort zone expands.

When our comfort zone expands in one area, it expands in others as well. When we succeed at something, our confidence and self-esteem increase.

I am willing to take on challenges.

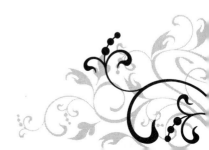

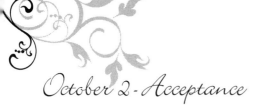

October 2 - Acceptance

Acceptance is simply seeing something exactly as it is and saying, *"That's the way it is."*

Acceptance is not approval, permission, agreement, sympathy, support, or even liking what it is.

When we accept, we relax; we let go.

Caregiving is about acceptance.

I accept things as they are.

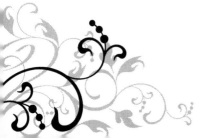

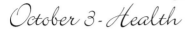

October 3 - Health

Our health, and the health of our loved-one, is more than the lack of illness. Health is aliveness, energy, joy, and love.

We can get better without ever getting sick.

Health is not just for the body. Health includes our mind and emotions. As caregivers, we must let our healthy energy flow in us, and through us.

I accept good health as the natural state of my being.

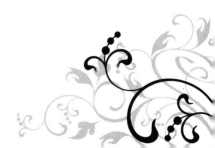

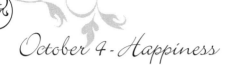

October 4 - Happiness

Happiness does not always come easily. It requires courage, grit, persistence, substance, and work.

Happiness takes practice, patience, and discipline.

It takes strength to be happy.

Be all that you can be. Join the happy.

I am surrounded by happiness and joy.

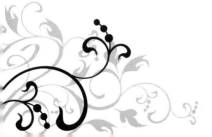

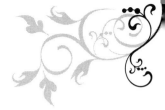

October 5 - Love

Caregiving is an act of love. When we reach out and give love unconditionally, focus on another's needs, love will return to us.

The attitude we cultivate will determine how the events of our lives affect us.

If we meet life with love, we will find love.

I rejoice in the love I have to share.

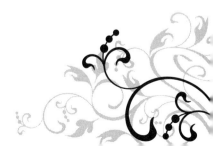

October 6 - Sacrifice

Few caregivers can perform superhumanly for years on end. The reality of undertaking sacrifice is that it almost always exacts some toll.

Without replenishing ourselves regularly, our capacity to keep giving is reduced.

We can alleviate the risk of becoming totally encumbered in caregiving by scheduling regular breaks from the job.

Today I will get more help and guidance.

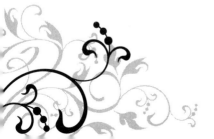

October 7 - Support

Choice and logistical support are important in caregiving; but so is emotional support.

Emotional support can take different forms: acknowledgment, compassion, and endorsement. We must reach out to others to share our burdens and sacrifices.

I am willing to let go of the struggle and ask for more help.

October 8 - Money

Money shapes or colors caregiving, as it does most other human endeavors. Money causes us to set limits on what we can do. It also forces us to prioritize.

We must learn to compromise and realize that caregiving may not necessarily be on our loved ones' terms, but rather our own.

I always get everything I need.

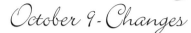

October 9 - Changes

We can expect changes and transitions for ourselves through the care-receiver's disease process.

The transitions from one caregiving stage to the next will take more time, energy, and resources.

We must be mindful of the ways in which we are growing as caregivers. We can see more clearly what is important and what is not.

I change my thinking with love.

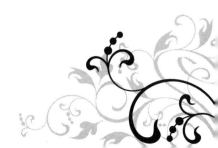

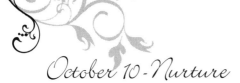

October 10 - Nurture

Through the caregiving process we try to understand our loved-one. We nurture what the care-receiver can still do.

We can never give up thinking about ways in which our loved-one can be stimulated, safe, and still feel a sense of purpose.

We must stay alert to recognize the clues for transitions that are taking place.

Harmony and peace surround me.

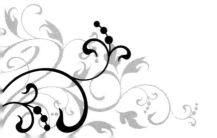

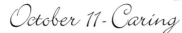

October 11 - Caring

We understand there is no perfect way to give care. We learn from others that some ways work better than others.

Each caregiver experiences caregiving uniquely. Being flexible while making adjustments for ourselves and the person in our care, throughout the caregiving process is very important.

Every day we must search for ways to help us remain enthusiastic about giving care.

I allow my love to touch others.

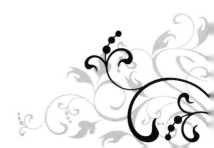

October 12 - Appreciation

We often focus upon what is wrong instead of what is right about ourselves and our style of caregiving. The consequences of such imbalance include pain and fear.

When we practice appreciation, we quiet poor self-judgment and criticism in ourselves.

Take a moment to accentuate the good instead of the bad.

I am very grateful to be exactly where I am today.

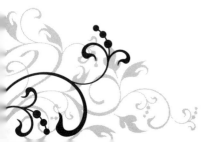

October 13 - Change

Outlining the steps we need to achieve our goals facilitates our ability to focus. Goal-oriented tasks, however small, give us the direction and purpose in caregiving.

We need to take simple and gradual steps to make lasting changes in our caregiving world. We often confuse change with giant leaps forward and overnight results. Caregiving is a long term process.

I trust the process of change.

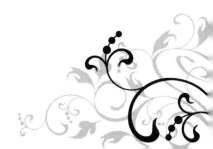

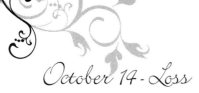

October 14 - Loss

Past memories of loss can stay with us like gaping wounds that never completely heal. The more we think about them, the more they feed our sense of failure, pain, and fears.

Living and working in regret is an unhealthy place to dwell.

I have come this far, and I am stronger for it.

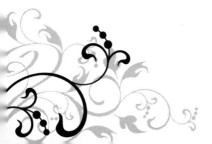

October 15 - Stress

Managing stress is an ongoing activity. If our loved-one's condition worsens, the stress felt by the caregiver is likely to grow.

We can do much to help ourselves. We can explore community services, and we must recognize our limitations, especially during a long period of intense care.

Without outside support, caregivers can develop stress-induced illnesses such as depression and anxiety.

I can handle all that is given to me today.

October 16 - Limits

There are times when caregivers will exercise nurture and authority. Sometimes setting limits and taking charge will be called for; other times, our loved-ones will need nurturing from us.

It probably feels more comfortable to be nurturing. It may not feel comfortable to be authoritative and taking charge.

Sometimes tough love is required.

I will take charge when I need to.

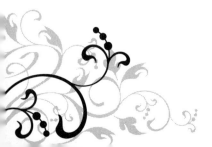

October 17 - Over-involvement

Over-involvement is a form of bargaining. It becomes dangerous when we fail to seek help when we should.

Over time, when emotional compensations begin to fail, other strong negative emotions emerge.

I choose to make my life light and enjoyable.

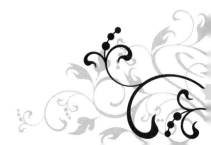

October 18 - Expectations

It is not an easy job to change our expectations or image of a person we have known for a lifetime. However, an examination of our beliefs about our care-receiver can give us new insights into interacting with loved-ones.

We can gain more control of the situation and can help the care-receiver to retain his/her capacity to reason, understand, and act appropriately as long as possible.

I will temper my expectations with reality.

October 19 - Understanding

We caregivers have a tendency to put pressure on ourselves. Lacking a full understanding of the physical causes of the illness and its impact on the care-receiver's functional capabilities, we hold ourselves responsible for our loved-one's failures.

Anger, guilt, frustration, and similar feelings can push us beyond our limits. We must understand this connection and prevent the negative consequences.

I know it's the condition, not me.

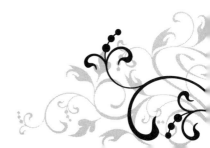

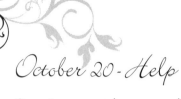

October 20 - Help

Caregivers must learn to solicit and accept the help of others during the course of the care-receiver's illness.

Those of us who find this difficult should examine our beliefs.

As the disease progresses, we will find ourselves shouldering increased responsibility for our loved-one.

I have faith and perseverance to become a better caregiver.

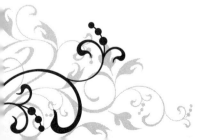

October 21 - Response

Caregivers can respond more appropriately to the care-receiver's problems when we identify the various reasons for their reactions.

The perceived problem may not always be the real problem. Beliefs and feelings about a problem can lead to interpretations, judgments, and reactions that can prevent us from successfully handling the situation.

I am guided by wisdom and love.

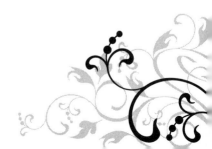

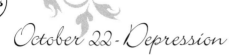

October 22 - Depression

Caregiving is associated with conditions that foster the development of depression and considerable levels of stress.

Our duties and responsibilities increase in proportion to the increasing dependency of loved-ones.

Recognizing the possibility that depression is developing is the first step toward treatment.

I am able to see the light.

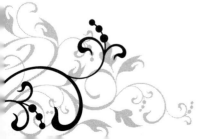

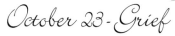

October 23 - Grief

Caregivers experience grief. Distinguishing depression from grief can be difficult since they both share some symptoms.

No matter how I feel today, I begin my day by letting go to a power greater than myself.

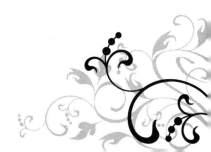

October 24 - Burden

Burden is a risk factor for depression. Caregiving burdens may include some or all of the following: cost, time, energy, anxiety, health problems, and social and psychological aspects of caregiving.

Higher levels of caregiver burden increase the risk of depression.

A positive outlook on life and the use of effective coping strategies are associated with less distress and burden.

I am open to feel all that there is — knowing that I can handle all that comes my way.

October 25 - Support

Caregivers need to develop avenues of social support. Social support refers to the parts of relationships that are positive and stress-reducing.

Social support reinforces our belief that others care about us.

We receive valuable feedback about how well we are coping.

It keeps us plugged in to the rest of the world.

I am willing to make changes.

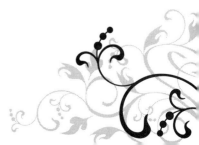

October 26 - Choice

Caregivers who perceive they have choices about care and caregiving will have more success adapting to the situation than caregivers who see no choices.

We have to nurture our coping resiliency to ward off depression.

I choose to enjoy being a caregiver.

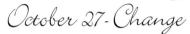

October 27 - Change

Loved-ones will change as will the relationship caregivers have with them.

We bring our own skills and resources to the caregiving situation.

Both the needs of the care-receiver and caregiver must be addressed.

Caregivers must assimilate information and knowledge to know how best to handle the situation.

I move forward without hesitation.

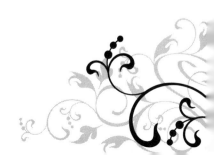

October 28 - Self-Talk

We engage in self-talk every day. It is important to pay close attention to how we think about and interpret daily stressors.

When we become aware of what we are saying to ourselves and how it influences our reactions to stress, we can be successful in managing stress.

Rational self-talk reflects our reality accurately and supports healthy functioning.

I handle all ideas with love and ease.

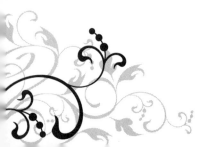

October 29 - Coping

For the most part, coping involves doing something to change what is stressful, or thinking differently about situations and events.

Changing a stressful situation may involve analyzing the problem and taking steps to deal directly with whatever is causing the stress.

Different stressors may call for different approaches.

I am aware of the stressful points in my life.

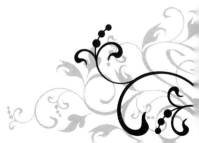

October 30 - Community Resources

The physical and mental strain placed on the caregiver can be significantly reduced if both family and community resources are sufficiently utilized.

Community resources become more important as we become more isolated and tired.

It is important for us to explore the resources available to us before our loved-one's condition progresses.

I listen to others and let them help me.

October 31 - Mistakes

None of us feels great when we make a mistake. However small, it can grate on us to no end. But mistakes can also be gifts, doorways to growth and wisdom.

There is no blueprint for being a caregiver. Mistakes can be excellent teachers who guide us along a bumpy road to a place of understanding.

When we make a mistake, we need to give ourselves permission to be open to the valuable lesson that will improve our lives.

I enjoy new ways of thinking.

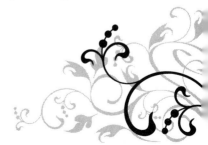

November 1 - Barriers

An ongoing problem for caregivers of mentally ill adults is the tension between treatment needs and legal barriers to care.

Family caregiving of persons with severe mental illness is often difficult and unrewarding.

Caregivers are forced to learn to deal both with the care-receiver's behaviors and with their own reactions. We must learn how and when.

I know when to say no.

November 2 - Thoughtfulness

Talk about the simple things can go a long way. When we care, we should show it.

Things as simple as a greeting card or something else inexpensive, yet meaningful, that sums up how we feel are all we need to make an impact and strengthen a relationship.

I rejoice in others' happiness.

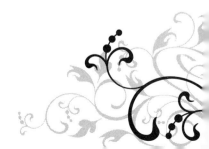

November 3 - Spoken Words

For most of us, our words are spoken without consciousness. We rarely stop to think about what we are saying.

Our thoughts and judgments roll off our tongues without a care for the damage or benefits they can produce.

To be a better caregiver, we need to speak words that will build self-esteem, self-confidence and build relationships.

My words are loving and kind.

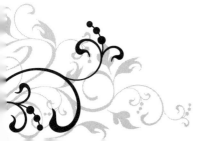

November 4 - Self-care

Taking care of ourselves will enable us to continue providing quality care to our loved-one.

To help cope with the demands of quality caregiving, we can:
- Set realistic goals.
- Learn more about caregiving and make learning an ongoing process.
- Do not confuse doing with caring.

I love and accept myself.

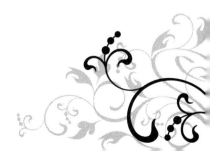

November 5 - Spirituality

Some caregivers may find it helpful to consider caregiving from a spiritual perspective. We try to find a deeper meaning beyond day-to-day tasks,

We think of what we are doing as a meaningful, rewarding experience rather than as simply a job or obligation.

We derive pleasure and satisfaction from caring for others.

My Higher Power guides me every day.

November 6 - Grief

Caregiver grief is a paradox — we are mourning the loss, while the person we are mourning stands in front of us.

Grieving both big and small losses means acknowledging that losses are happening. It is important that we nurture the life that remains.

It means finding joy in the present moment and acknowledgment of a past that is gone.

I live today as I want to remember my life.

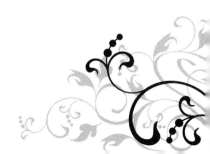

November 7 - Remembering

Things do not always turn out the way we want. Life can take strange turns that are out of our control. When thoughts come up that remind us of times when people, places and things did not work out in a positive way, stop and sit back and take some quiet time.

Caregiving is a process. We have to remember the good that we have done, the kindnesses given and the love shown to and by others.

I listen to my inner voice with a new trust today.

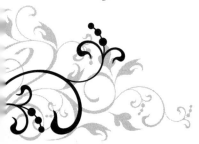

November 8 - Reactions

Our reactions to our caregiving role and to the care-receiver, both positive and negative, are a function of both our kinship relationship and our loved-one's personal characteristics and illness history.

Caregiving stress also varies as a function of physical energy and other role demands concordant with our age or a particular stage in our life cycle.

I relax, knowing that all the details of the day will fall into place.

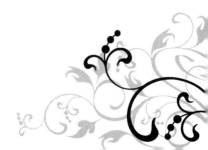

November 9 - Decisions

Deciding what is best for our loved-one and ourselves requires us to be realistic and not emotional.

We cannot deceive ourselves or let feelings of guilt interfere with an honest appraisal of our options.

We cannot make decisions lightly — or alone. We should involve our loved-one as well as other family members and members of the caregiving team.

I am a decisive person. I follow through on my promises.

November 10 - Perspective

As dementia or Alzheimer's disease progresses, the care-receiver becomes more confused and experiences personality and behavior changes. He or she will require more care, which can become increasingly difficult and exhausting for the caregiver.

Keeping a positive perspective and a good sense of humor can help us cope with challenging times ahead.

I will celebrate the good things in my life.

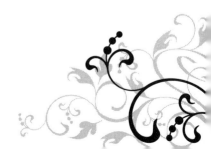

November 11 - Duty

When we become caregivers, there is no rule that we have to be the sole caregiver indefinitely.

When caregiving duties become more than we can bear or a family member requires medical attention or constant care that we simply can't provide, it's time to research other options. In the long run, this is best for the caregiver and care-receiver.

I will receive fully that which is offered today.

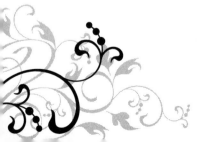

November 12 - Life

Though we may feel energetic and in super health now, caring for an aged loved-one can provide a sobering lesson that life can change in a flash — and often in ways we would have never chosen.

Instead of worrying about what could or may happen, caregivers who have been there before us, recommend heeding the lesson to prepare for our own future and to appreciate and make the most of our lives now.

I will take care of my life today.

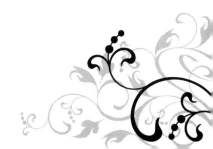

November 13 - Support

When the stresses of caregiving start to get to us, nothing helps like talking over our troubles with a sympathetic friend.

Bottling up our emotions can lead to caregiver burnout. Talking frees us up; sharing our feelings and fears reduces our feeling of being overburdened.

There is no need to struggle. I will let others help me.

November 14 - Dreams

When caregiving interferes with our goals and dreams, it is important to take pleasure in the little things that are in our immediate environment.

Every day, we have to try and find something to celebrate, something to be happy about.

We must learn to enjoy the simple things.

Today holds a special promise for me.

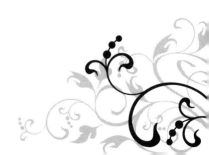

November 15 - Feelings

Feelings are feelings — nothing more, nothing less.

Having negative feelings about caregiving doesn't make us bad caregivers. It's natural to have conflicted feelings about caregiving.

The way we act on our feelings can turn into a bad situation, especially if anger and guilt take over.

We must acknowledge our feelings, accept them, and then move on.

My courage will conquer any ill feelings I have today.

November 16 - Calmness

Deep breathing helps calm people (caregivers) down. When in distress, most people breathe rapidly but shallowly.

To dissipate stress:
1. Empty your lungs by breathing out.
2. Take a deep breath; feel the air flowing through your nose to the abdomen.
3. Hold your breath for a few seconds.
4. Breathe out slowly through your mouth.
5. Repeat steps 1-4 ten times.

Today I will weigh my behavior carefully.

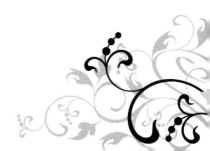

November 17 - Feelings

It is unlikely that either the caregiver or care-receiver planned to spend their later years in a caregiving situation. These changes in lifestyle, economic security, responsibilities, and relationships are accompanied by emotional responses.

These feelings are particularly troublesome because of the guilt which often accompanies them.

Ignoring our feelings does not make them go away.

I will accept variations from my planned life with gratitude.

November 18 - Conflict

When our feelings are not recognized or when they are denied and unresolved, they can lead to conflict in relationships and to physical and emotional problems for the individuals involved.

Caregivers can cope by accepting and acknowledging their feelings; and by becoming aware of how the care-receiver is coping and what this is doing in the relationship.

I will open myself fully in order to hear clearly.

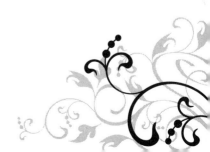

November 19 - Behavior

When a disrupting behavior is seen as an expression of an individual's discomfort over loss of control or the fight to regain some control, we need to respond to the underlying cause, rather than to the behavior.

The key to change is to allow the individual to maintain control in every way possible; reinforcing self-esteem.

I will exercise my power to behave well.

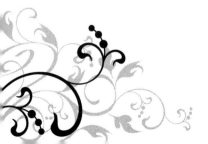

November 20 - Expectations

In many caregiver cases, role expectations are not clear, or people do not agree about what is expected. This can be a stressful situation.

The role of caregiver often creates conflicts within a person because of personal expectations about appropriate ways to perform as a spouse or adult child.

New roles and rules must be defined and expectations clarified within the individual and within the family.

I am open to new beginnings.

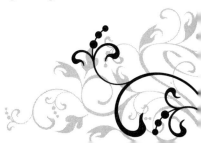

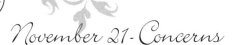

November 21 - Concerns

Common emotions expressed by caregivers are worry, fear, embarrassment, shame, grief, anger, depression, helplessness, and guilt.

Caregivers worry their best efforts are not sufficient.

We are fearful not only for the fate of a loved-one, but also for our own future.

I won't get trapped today by a negative attitude.

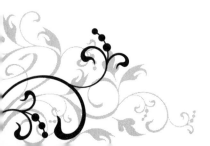

November 22 - Feelings

Caregivers should be aware that our own behaviors can affect the behavior of the care-receiver.

Suppressed feelings may be perceived by the care-receiver, and many times it is these feelings that bring on problem behaviors.

Caregivers must learn skills in managing annoying behaviors.

I have the personal power to influence my day.

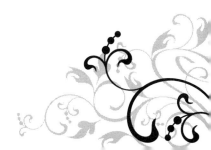

November 23 - Manipulation

The greatest amount of manipulation is done by care-receivers who are struggling to retain some control over the world around them.

Changes in the way each person handles life come slowly.

It is important to help the manipulator use more acceptable methods to let others know of their desires and needs.

I stand in truth.

November 24 - Anger

Suppressed anger, especially if it is just under the surface, can cause real problems in caring for family members. It is okay to be angry. It is what we do with that anger that is important.

Often suppressed anger will show itself in impatience or irritability towards the care-receiver. Also, feelings of guilt in the caregiver are often really anger turned inwards.

I am in charge of my emotions. I can control my feelings.

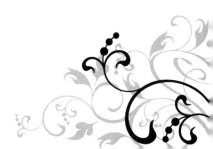

November 25 - Reminiscence

Reminiscence is a way of reliving, re-experiencing or savoring events of the past that are personally significant.

It can help the care-receiver to remember that his or her life has been of value, even if at present it no longer seems important.

Reminiscence helps the care-receiver to maintain self-esteem and reinforce a sense of identity; feel a sense of achievement and pleasure; and cope with stresses related to the aging process.

I will look to this day with wonder and trust.

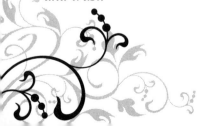

November 26 - Family

Family members may have difficulty with communication because they take each other for granted or have grown away from each other. In some families, members have never known very much about the real feelings and values of each other.

Families who want to draw together for decision making in support of a loved-one may need to develop new communication skills and styles.

I will be alert today to the needs of my family.

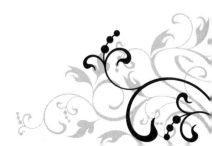

November 27 - Decisions

Decision making in stressful situations is difficult. Intuitive ways of deciding often fail because of the complexity of the situation and the need for several people to take action together. However, the issues may be too important for a *"best-guess"* approach.

I will look for the opportunities to share decision making.

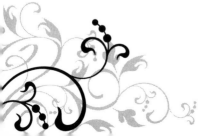

November 28 - Awareness

Awareness of our loved-one's medical condition will make us more nimble through the medical minefield.

We can never really know how the illness will affect everyone until we're in the middle of it, which is why becoming aware is such an important task.

I release the old and welcome the new.

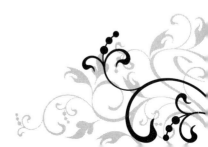

November 29 - Confusion

Confusion is not a *"normal"* change that occurs with aging. Confusion can result from many potentially treatable causes such as infection, poor nutrition, depression, undiagnosed illness, or in appropriate use of medications.

As a caregiver, we must press health professionals to consider confusion seriously and to look for causes which may be treatable.

I see clearly and move forward without hesitation.

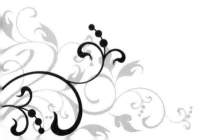

November 30 - Relationships

Personal relationships and daily interactions of all kinds are more satisfying when the people, both caregivers and care-receivers, are able to understand each other's viewpoints and to take in the other's perspective.

I will look for beauty in a friend; and I will find it.

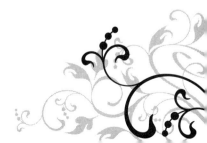

December 1 - Memory

At times, we can all be forgetful. We can help improve memory skills of the care-receiver by tactfully making some suggestions, by giving presents (calendars, photo albums, etc.) that can be used as reminders.

We must recognize when people are tired, sick, or tense, and avoid taxing their memory at that time.

A new set of experiences awaits me today.

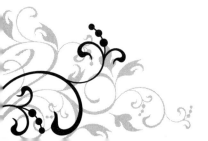

December 2 - Legalities

Generally, adults should have the right to maintain their independence and their dignity in every way possible. As our loved-one ages and becomes more impaired, family members and caregivers may best protect them by taking only legal steps that will provide needed support without taking over responsibilities that the individual is still able to manage.

I will not overstep my bounds.

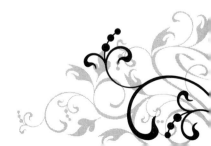

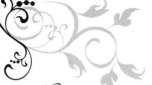

December 3 - Sleep

Periods of relaxation during the day can help compensate for some loss of sleep and can improve our ability to cope with stress.

Relaxation techniques can also be used to induce sleep more quickly when there is opportunity for it.

I am fulfilled. Life agrees with me.

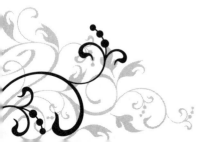

December 4 - Control

If we do not assert our own rights, others may be managing us.

We must think about our expectations for our daily lives. Each of us has different views about what is most important.

We must learn to accept what we cannot change or have no control over.

I look ahead freely.

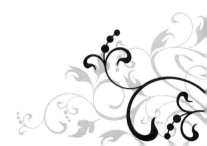

December 5 - Words

Putting our thoughts into spoken words will sometimes clarify them for us. Talking to a good friend or counselor may help to put our situation into perspective or to visualize new solutions.

Talk to someone who is willing to listen.

Sharing my feelings strengthens me and heals my wounds.

December 6 - Reflections

After a disturbing or frustrating experience with a care-receiver, we can take a moment to reflect on our previous accomplishments as a caregiver.

We can maintain a more positive mental balance when we can laugh at ourselves, and forgive ourselves for not being perfect.

I move into my greater good. I am secure.

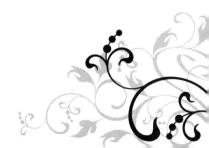

December 7 - Future

Caregivers must plan for the future. The time will come when our caregiving situation will no longer exist.

The planning process will give us mental relief and pleasure now.

It will also make the transition easier for us when this change comes into our lives.

Every person and every situation, adds to my success.

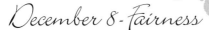

December 8 - Fairness

Life isn't fair. Life is just life. When we realize the fact that life isn't fair, it keeps us from feeling sorry for ourselves.

Just because life isn't fair doesn't mean we shouldn't do everything in our power to improve our own lives or our care-receiver's life.

Pity is a self-defeating emotion that does nothing for anyone, except to make everyone feel worse than they already do.

My life is unfolding exactly as it should.

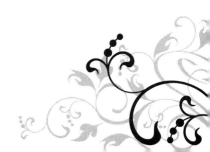

December 9 - Review

We should periodically review our commitment to being a caregiver.

Caregiving has the greatest chance of being sustained when there is lots of support.

Upon review, we may need to redefine our role as caregiver. We may need to enlist additional help. Ultimately this can benefit both the caregiver and the care-receiver.

Confidence will come with my healthy self-acceptance.

December 10 - Transformations

One of the predictors of our future is our past. If we look at our family relationships before a (medical) crisis, we will get a glimpse of what our caregiving relationships will probably resemble.

When family relationships are characterized by mutual misgivings and mistrust, caregiving will often be characterized the same way. There is usually not a major transformation in attitudes and behaviors just because a loved-one has a chronic condition.

I am courageous and independent.

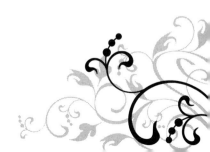

December 11 - Optimism

Not everyone is a cheery, optimistic person. However, practicing cautious optimism will carry us through the rough spots.

Reasonably optimistic caregivers keep the daily ups and downs in perspective and their emotional reactions under control.

Joy, love, peace. I rejoice in life.

December 12 - Burden

While a primary caregiver can be expected to feel the most burdened, other family members are affected by the changes that accompany taking care of a loved-one.

I let go of everything I no longer need.

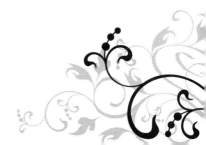

December 13 - Research

Caregiving can be a negative influence on our physical, psychological, and emotional well-being.

More research is needed in terms of what can be done to help caregivers manage our tasks efficiently and satisfactorily and at the same time maintain our own health, finances, and well being.

I can look around me and be thankful.

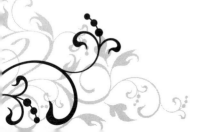

December 14 - Demands

The crunch of caregiver demands frequently leads to depression, anxiety, and a feeling of helplessness. Caregiver overload is especially common among the "*sandwich*" generation, or those caring for aging parents along with their own children.

A geriatric care manager can help ease this burden by offering counseling or recommending a family counselor.

I can teach myself patience.

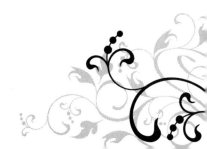

December 15 - Spirituality

Consider that perhaps the basic principle of spirituality is that our problems are the best places to practice keeping our hearts open.

When we accept our problems (especially in caregiving) as inevitable, natural, and even an important part of life – we will discover that life can be more of a dance and less of a fight.

In caregiving, go with the flow.

I trust the universe. Life supports me.

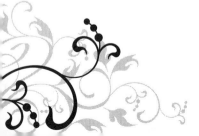

December 16 - Responsibilities

Caregiving often comes with new responsibilities and unfamiliar tasks, yet most caregivers never receive training.

A living will, healthcare power of attorney, and plan for after care (funeral arrangements) can help ensure peace of mind for the ill person as well as you, the caregiver.

I will persevere and find completion in today's tasks.

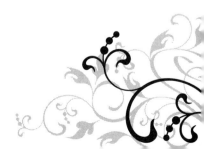

December 17 - End-of-Life

Caregiving for someone at the end of life can be a challenging, but rewarding experience.

Caregiving at the end of life may bring about many different feelings — it will be important for us to care for ourselves and ask for help when we need it.

I will rest from my thoughts.

December 18 - Depression

Regardless of the cause of depression, the result is the same. It robs people of the joy of life and can lead to other health problems.

Treatment for depression is necessary.

I will turn my attention to the world outside myself today.

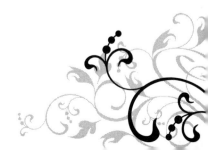

December 19 – Positive Reinforcement

It's easy to complain and whine when things are not going just right. This is especially true when we are overwhelmed and tired.

But instead of complaining when things go wrong, we can try praising our loved-one when things go right. Chances are the care-receiver wants to please us and will appreciate the encouragement.

I will be glad today for the sun's rays.

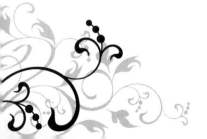

December 20 - Fear

Psychologists like to say that our fear means:

Fantasized
Experiences
Appearing
Real

All fear is self-created by imagining some negative outcome in the future.

Take a caregiving leap of faith, and trust your intuition and plunge in.

I will face my fears and be as strong as I need to be.

December 21 - Quality

Caregivers have the ability to transform seemingly insignificant situations into something enjoyable, meaningful, and memorable because of their conscious thinking and actions.

Caregivers can constantly enrich the lives of care-receivers by introducing significance, uniqueness, and stimulation into every day experiences.

Today offers me a miracle.

December 22 - Guidance

We can start our caregiving day over anytime that we choose just by a change of attitude.

If things are not going our way, we can pause and ask for guidance and positive energy and begin again.

If something happens that is disappointing or unpleasant, we do not need to let it spoil our whole day.

Today is wide open. All around me help is available.

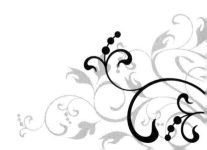

December 23 - Feelings

Sometimes caregivers might have to act *"as if"* to push beyond feelings, to get to the other side of them where we really want to be.

There are times when it is not appropriate to act how we really feel.

We might have to save those feelings and deal with them later in a more healthy and appropriate way.

Today, I will take time to the smell the roses.

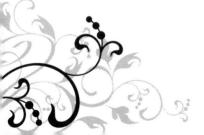

December 24 - Faith

There comes a time when we might be tired and weary and wonder why we are caregivers. There comes a time when all the work that we have done seems in vain.

The road ahead looks long, and there seems to be no end in sight.

Have faith.

I believe in better days.

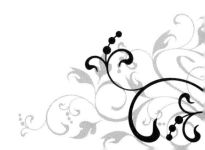

December 25 - Reality

When we project our caregiving fears into the future, we are living in a world that we are creating in our minds.

Reality is here and now. If we keep our minds here and now, we will have the energy to do the work that needs to be done.

I am grounded and look forward to challenges.

December 26 - Past History

We can't un-ring the bell. All that happened before this very second, is the past.

What is important is that we know right now that yesterday has no power over us, unless we let it.

Let yesterday serve as a light on all the caregiving lessons we no longer have to go through again.

I willingly forgive myself and others.

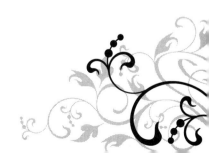

December 27 - Miracles

There are miracles in this day just waiting to be discovered. There are miracles at every corner.

There is a miracle in helping my loved-one, a miracle of forgiveness, a miracle of love.

I am in the right place, at the right time.

December 28 - Coping

If we view something as a problem, then it has meaning. If we can find other ways to think about the situation, the problem can be reframed and viewed differently.

Caregiving stress can be reduced by practicing different coping methods.

I choose to relax and live fully.

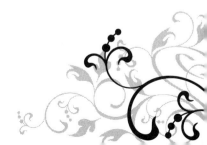

December 29 – Help

The family, and in particular, the primary caregiver, must learn to accept help. The burden of caregiving can otherwise cause serious problems and alienate us from friends and family who want to share the caregiving role.

Without help from others, the burden of care can become overwhelming.

Today I will slow down and seek out answers.

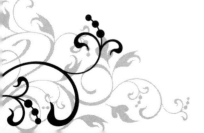

December 30 - Conflicts

Family conflicts interfere with social support. If family members drop out of the social support role, it may be difficult to replace them.

Conflict involving family members' attitudes and behaviors toward the caregiver has been found to be closely associated with caregiver depression.

I am letting go of all judgments.

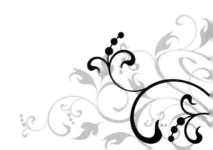

December 31 - Joy

We have come such a long way to get to this point in our lives. We have traveled many miles of the caregiving journey — including sorrow and happiness, pain and joy, defeat and victory.

Let go of the burdens and live with the joys of being a caregiver.

And now that the year is just about over, tomorrow, turn the page back to January 01 and let's start anew.

I am free.

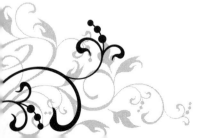

Topic Index

Abuse ....May 28
Acceptance..............Apr. 26, Aug. 13
Acknowledgment...May 21
Action ....Jan. 26
Adversity ....Sep. 3
Advice......................Jun. 27
Affection ....Mar. 13
Affirmation ....Jan. 2, Mar. 1
Anger........................Mar. 29, Apr. 17, Jul. 8, Jul. 26, Nov. 24
Anxiety.....................Feb. 23
Appreciation ....Oct. 12
Approval ....Apr. 27
Assessments...........Aug. 2
Assistance ....Jun. 10
Attitude....................Jan. 8, Apr. 14, Aug. 16, Sep. 7, Nov. 24
Awareness...............Nov. 28
Balance ....Apr. 10, May 31, Jul. 16, Jul. 29, Aug. 30, Sep. 30

Topic Index

Bargaining .... Oct. 17
Barriers .... Nov. 1
Behavior .... Nov. 19
Belief .... Jan. 17, Sep. 15
Benefits .... Aug. 19
Blessings .... Feb. 27
Boundaries .... May 30
Breathing .... Jan. 6, Jul. 25
Burden .... Oct. 24, Dec. 12
Burnout .... Apr. 26, Aug. 13
Calmness .... Nov. 16
Care Plan .... Aug. 11
Caring .... Oct. 11
Challenges .... Feb. 17, May 15
Change .... Mar. 12, Jun. 14, Sep. 19, Oct. 9,
                             Oct. 13, Oct. 27
Checklist .... Apr. 21
Choice .... Apr. 6, Oct. 26, Aug. 15

Topic Index

Comfort Zone	Oct. 1
Communication	Jan. 13, Mar. 16, Mar. 31, Jun. 28, Jul. 19, Aug. 22, Sep. 5
Compliments	Mar. 1
Concerns	Nov. 21
Confidence	Jan. 21, Sep. 28
Conflict	Sep. 10, Nov. 18, Dec. 30
Confusion	Nov. 29
Consistency	Nov. 11
Control	Dec. 4
Coping	Mar. 25, Oct. 29, Dec. 28
Counseling	Mar. 8
Creativity	Jan. 11, Aug. 24, Sep. 2
Criticism	Apr. 20
Death	Feb. 16, Aug. 1
Decisions	Mar. 24, Apr. 1, Jun. 11, Jun. 19, Jul. 28, Nov. 9, Nov. 27
Demands	Dec. 14
Depression	Apr. 3, Nov. 22, Dec. 18

Topic Index

Disagreements .... Jun. 22
Distractions .... Sep. 23
Doubt .... Sep. 27
Dreams .... Nov. 14
Duty .... Nov. 11
Education .... May 16
Effectiveness .... Sep. 26
Encouragement ...... May 23, Jun. 23, Sep. 16
End-of-life .... Mar. 9
Energy .... May 2
Excitement .... May 1
Exercise .... Jan. 28, Jul. 18, Sep. 29
Expectations .... Feb. 24, Apr. 12, Oct. 18, Nov. 20
Experience .... Feb. 21
Fairness .... Dec. 18
Faith .... Dec. 24
Family .... Mar. 26, Nov. 26
Family Issues .... Jun. 6

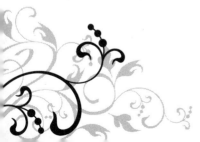

Topic Index

Fear	Jan. 7, Mar. 22, Jun. 20, Dec. 20
Feedback	Jan. 12
Feelings	Feb. 2, Mar. 20, Jun. 13, Jun. 25, Nov. 15, Nov. 17, Nov. 22, Dec. 23
Finances	Jul. 23
Financial Stress	Jun. 8
Flexibility	Jan. 26, May 24
Forgiveness	Jan. 29, Jul. 30
Friendships	Feb. 3, Feb. 11, Mar. 2, Jul. 4, Aug. 27
Frustration	May 6, Jul. 22, Aug. 19
Future	Jul. 6, Dec. 7
Gifts	Jun. 17
Giving in	Apr. 16
Goals	Jul. 17
Gratitude	Jan. 15, May 8, Aug. 20
Grief	Jan. 30, Mar. 7, May 29, Aug. 6, Oct. 23, Nov. 6
Guidance	Dec. 22

Topic Index

Guilt..........................Feb. 29, Mar. 23, Apr. 23
Habits.......................Sep. 4
Happiness ....Jan. 10, Jul. 3, Oct. 4
Health ....Jan. 3, Mar. 4, Mar. 5, Sep. 12, Oct. 3
Help ....Apr. 24, Jun. 4, Jul 20, Aug. 3, Aug. 15, Sep. 18, Sep. 21, Oct. 20, Dec. 29
Helplessness...........Mar. 14
Honesty...................Aug. 12
Hope........................Jun. 18
Humility ....Aug. 4
Humor.....................Apr. 8, Aug. 8
Image.......................Jun. 16
Imagination.............Mar. 3
Imperfection ....Feb. 4
Independence.........Mar. 15
Information.............Mar. 6
Inner Peace ....Feb. 7

Topic Index

Inner Self	Mar. 18
Integrity	Aug. 18
Intentions	Aug. 29
Intervention	May 25
Involvement	May 20
Isolation	Apr. 30
Joy	Dec. 31
Kindness	Feb. 18, May 9
Knowledge	May 4, Aug. 17
Laughter	Jan. 4, Feb. 1
Learning	Jul. 7
Legalities	Dec. 2
Life	Nov. 12
Limitations	Sep. 14
Limits	Jun. 12, Oct. 16
Listening	Sep. 17
Loss	Oct. 14
Love	Jun. 15, Oct. 5
Luck	May 12

Topic Index

Management..........Apr. 11

Manipulation ....Nov. 23

Memory ....Dec. 1

Miracles ....Dec. 27

Mistakes..................Oct. 31

Moderation ....Jan. 25

Money ....Oct. 8

Motivation...............May 13

Nurture....................Oct. 10

Obstacles ....Feb. 12, May 18

Optimism.................Dec. 11

Options....................Jun. 1

Organization...........Apr. 2, Jul. 1

Overcoming ....Feb. 19

Pain ....Mar. 19

Parents.....................Jul. 24

Past..........................Mar. 28, Dec. 26

Patience ....Jan. 27

Topic Index

Perfection	Apr. 19, Sep. 9
Personality Styles	Jun. 26
Perspective	Feb. 5, Nov. 10
Planning	Feb. 13, Apr. 22, May 27
Positive	Dec. 19
Positive Attitude	Jan. 24, Feb. 14
Possibilities	Jan. 1
Power	Feb. 9
Praise	Feb. 26
Prayer	Jul. 12
Preparation	Jan. 19
Pressure	Jan. 23, Sep. 1
Problem Solve	Apr. 15
Problems	April 5
Purpose	Aug. 14
Quality	Dec. 21
Reactions	Jan. 9, Nov. 8
Reality	May 11, Jun. 30, Dec. 25
Recreation	Aug. 28

Topic Index

Reflection .... Feb. 10, Apr. 13, Dec. 6
Relationships .... May 7, Sep. 8, Nov. 30
Release .... Jul. 29
Relief .... Feb. 22
Remembering .... Nov. 7
Reminiscence .... Mar. 30, Nov. 25
Research .... Dec. 13
Resources .... Oct. 30
Respite .... Jan. 20, Apr. 9, Apr. 29, Jun. 2, Jun. 24
Response .... Oct. 21
Responsibilities ..... Jul. 15, Dec. 16
Review .... Dec. 9
Rewards .... May 22
Role Reversal .... Jun. 5
Routine .... Apr. 7
Sacrifice .... Oct. 6
Self-awareness ...... Jul. 12

Topic Index

Self-care	Feb. 8, Jun. 21, Jul. 21, Nov. 4
Self-control	Jan. 5
Self-talk	Aug. 25, Oct. 28
Serenity	Feb. 6
Sharing	Aug. 31
Siblings	Jul. 11
Skills	May 5
Sleep	Jul. 5, Dec. 3
Spirituality	Nov. 5, Dec. 15
Strengths	Feb. 28, Jul. 9
Stress	Jan. 14, Mar. 10, Jun. 3, Aug. 9, Sep. 6, Sep. 13, Oct. 15
Stress Mgt.	May 26
Stress Relief	Apr. 28
Styles	Jun. 9
Success	May 3, Aug. 21
Support	Feb. 25, Mar. 21, Apr. 4, May 17, Jun. 7, Jul. 14, Jul. 31, Aug. 23, Oct. 7, Oct. 25, Nov. 13

Topic Index

Tact .... Aug. 26
Teamwork .... Jan. 18
Tenacity .... Feb. 20
Thoughtfulness .... Nov. 2
Time .... Jan. 31
Timing .... Jul. 13
Touch .... May 19, Aug. 7
Toxic People .... Jul. 10
Traits .... May 10
Transformation ...... Sep. 22, Dec. 10
Trust .... Jul. 27
Truth .... Feb. 15
Understanding .... Oct. 19
Validation .... Jun. 29
Visualization .... Jan. 22, Sep. 25
Words .... Nov. 3, Dec. 5
Workload .... Mar. 11, Apr. 18
Worry .... Mar. 27, May 14

Notes

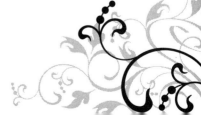

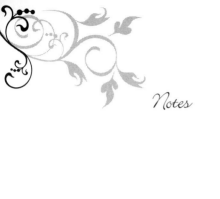

Notes

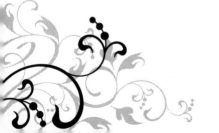